Mobilizing the Community for Better Health

Mobilizing the Community for Better Health

What the Rest of America Can Learn from Northern Manhattan

EDITED BY

ALLAN J. FORMICOLA

AND

LOURDES HERNÁNDEZ-CORDERO

Columbia University Press   *New York*

Columbia University Press
Publishers Since 1893
New York   Chichester, West Sussex
Copyright © 2011 Columbia University Press
All rights reserved

Library of Congress Cataloging-in-Publication Data

Mobilizing the community for better health : what the rest of America can learn from
Northern Manhattan / edited by Allan J. Formicola and Lourdes Hernández-Cordero.
    p. ; cm.
  Includes bibliographical references and index.
  ISBN 978-0-231-15166-5 (cloth : alk. paper)—ISBN 978-0-231-15167-2 (pbk. : alk.
paper)—ISBN 978-0-231-52527-5 (ebook)
    1. Community health services—New York (State)—New York.   2. Hospital and
community—New York (State)—New York.   3. Medical policy—New York (State)—New
York.   4. Health promotion—New York (State)—New York.   5. Health services
accessibility—New York (State)—New York.   I. Formicola, Allan J.   II. Hernández-
Cordero, Lourdes.
    [DNLM: 1. Columbia University.   2. Community Health Services—methods—New
York City.   3. Community-Institutional Relations—New York City.   4. Health Plan
Implementation—methods—New York City.   5. Health Policy—New York City.   6. Health
Promotion—organization & administration—New York City.   7. Health Services
Accessibility—organization & administration—New York City.   WA 546 AN7]

  RA395.A4N744 2010
  362.12097471—dc22

                                                                    2010026496

Columbia University Press books are printed on permanent and durable acid-free paper.
This book is printed on paper with recycled content.
Printed in the United States of America

c 10 9 8 7 6 5 4 3 2 1
p 10 9 8 7 6 5 4 3 2 1

This book is dedicated to Dr. Henrie Treadwell and to the people of Washington Heights/Inwood and Harlem.

Dr. Treadwell was the guiding light for the Community Voices program. She set the pace for all of the participating sites. Dr. Treadwell infused the "heart and soul" into Community Voices. As the program director of the W. K. Kellogg Foundation's Community Voices: Health Care for the Underserved program, she brought together a supportive team to assist us in meeting and exceeding the goals of our projects. It was especially gratifying to work with her, as she was a motivator, taskmaster, and model for each of us working on the initiative. Dr. Treadwell is a tireless advocate for those in society who are often called the voiceless. Through this program she gave them a voice and continues to do so now at the Primary Care Center at Morehouse School of Medicine.

Washington Heights/Inwood and Harlem, the sites for the Northern Manhattan Community Voices Collaborative, provided an invigorating environment for the work of the collaborative and the inspiration for the work accomplished. The two communities are blessed with many dedicated leaders in community-based organizations and in the clergy. Along with their locally elected officials, they opened doors that permitted the two communities to make enormous advances for their residents. The communities are diverse and provide an exceptional setting for the institutions of which they are a part. They are truly the melting pot that makes the United States the envy of the world.

Contents

Contents

List of Figures

List of Tables

Foreword

Out of a belief that the best solutions to improving health in underserved communities can come from the insights and wisdom of the residents of those communities, the W. K. Kellogg Foundation launched a $55 million national initiative in 1998 called Community Voices: Health Care for the Underserved. Bringing the diverse voices of an entire community to the table to promote action around improving health was the core strategy of the initiative, which funded thirteen sites across the nation. The foundation wanted to create models responsive to local interests and raise them up as national models to help address the crisis in health care and the growing number of uninsured, underinsured, and underserved citizens. These dynamic "learning laboratories" were local collaborations among institutions, government, and community, supported under the premise that members of underserved communities, when equipped with information, tools, and resources, can and should contribute to reorienting the health care delivery system.

As one of the largest initiatives to be undertaken in the W. K. Kellogg Foundation's history, Community Voices was a six-year investment that affirmed our dedication to some precious principles—our belief in community-driven change, and in partnerships strengthened by the glue of collaboration. The work of these grantees extended what we understood then and reinforces what we know today about the process of change—that it requires both top-down and bottom-up movements of thought and action. Engagement at the community level must inform regional, state, and national dialogue; and policy endeavors in the halls of government must take into account the voices of those who benefit from services, or suffer from their lack—voices that historically have been excluded.

To explore ways to expand coverage and access for underserved populations and broaden the definition of health, grantees formed coalitions and working groups of all shapes and sizes to engage in creative problem solving. In New York, it was the Northern Manhattan Community Voices Collaborative (NMCVC) that signed on to create locally generated solutions to improve health care access and quality. As in the other communities, the NMCVC benefited from leadership with the passion, willingness, and vision to tackle making their local health care system more responsive to community residents.

In *Mobilizing the Community for Better Health: What the Rest of America Can Learn from Northern Manhattan*, the authors share tales from their ten-year journey to join thirty-five community organizations and health care providers to improve the overall health of their community. Serving a largely Dominican/Latino and African American population in Washington Heights/Inwood and central Harlem, the initiative was led by the Columbia University College of Dental Medicine, Harlem Hospital Center, and Alianza Dominicana.

Dr. Allan Formicola and Dr. Lourdes J. Hernández-Cordero and the other contributors to this volume describe how the NMCVC transformed the skills and outlook of individuals who worked in the collaboration; improved the health of individuals who benefited from the programs; and increased the capacity of partner organizations. They share how community health workers contributed to making health care appropriate and accessible in ways other members of the health workforce could not; how they began to raise access to oral and mental health services to a par with primary care access; and why health policy efforts must be integrated into all program initiatives if they are to sustain themselves. While not all of these efforts met with the same degree of success, they provide engaging stories with powerful lessons for anyone interested in reducing health disparities. This readable and practical supplemental text for faculty and students in public health and health administration courses is a valuable guide for community-based organizations, service providers, government officials, professional organizations, advocates, and policy makers working to address today's realities of health care reform.

At a time when our nation nears the possibility of joining other developed nations in the world by providing some form of universal access to health care, the authors share successful strategies for solving problems that continue to daunt decision makers in board rooms, public institutions, and the halls of government. In essence, this book reveals much about the potential of communities to reorient our nation's health systems to meet the needs of everyone, with lessons that many decision makers need to hear and heed.

Gail C. Christopher
Vice President for Programs
W. K. Kellogg Foundation

Acknowledgments

Preparing this book has been an important capstone to the Northern Manhattan Community Voices Collaborative. We did not believe we could just close the door on the initiative and leave unsaid the many challenges and accomplishments of all of the wonderful people who in one way or another worked in the collaborative over a ten-year period. When we started to outline the book and begin the process it seemed overwhelming. In reflecting back over the process of writing the book, we first have to acknowledge the efforts of two key collaborators, Nancy Bruning and Yisel Alonzo. Nancy, an experienced editor and author, came aboard to help us organize the effort and to work with all of the chapter authors in editing their drafts. She kept the process moving along and prevented us from bogging down. Yisel prepared all of the Northern Manhattan Community Voices Collaborative files so that information was retrievable. The enthusiasm of Nancy and Yisel made the job of preparing the book much easier for us!

We thank the W. K. Kellogg Foundation for having the confidence in us to award us the first grant of $4.5 million and the follow-up grant of $1 million to complement our efforts with policy work. We acknowledge with great appreciation Barbara Sabol, the Kellogg program officer who oversaw the Community Voices initiative. Henrie Treadwell was the Kellogg project director for the initiative, and her guiding light moved us to dedicate this book to her.

We also acknowledge her help in gaining a Kellogg Foundation grant for $1 million for start-up funds for the Adair Center when funding for charitable efforts dried up for projects in New York City as it was directed toward the aftermath of 9/11. The Community Voices national program office under Henrie Treadwell's leadership provided much technical assistance for all of the thirteen participating sites through national meetings, individual meetings with each site, and evaluations of our progress. We were fortunate to also have the assistance of Marguerite Ro, one of the Kellogg Foundation consultants for the Community Voices initiative who was also a faculty member at Columbia. Her advice was always solid and helped us during the years of the project. We thank Gail Christopher at the foundation who, in her role as vice president for health, wrote the foreword for the book.

We also acknowledge other funders who provided direct support for the initiatives described in the book. The American Legacy Foundation joined the Community Voices initiative, and we thank the foundation for the $800,000 grant to carry out the Tobacco initiative described in chapter 6. New York State provided funds to Alianza Dominicana for the facilitated enrollment work cited in chapter 3. The Primary Care Development Corporation and its executive director Ronda Kotelchuck are acknowledged for a $400,000 grant for the Thelma Adair Center, and the Empire State Development Corporation is acknowledged for providing $2 million in construction funds for the Center (chapter 13). Columbia University College of Physicians and Surgeons and the College of Dental Medicine are recognized for sustaining the Adair Center financially during the first seven years of its existence and for the work it has accomplished in transferring the facility to a Federally Qualified Health Center, the Ryan Center. The Health Resources Services Administration provided the funding for the SASA project (chapter 7), and the Greater New York Hospital Association provided a grant for the work that the Northern Manhattan Community Voices Collaborative did on the HITE program (chapter 8). The Community DentCare Network has attracted many funders. A $1 million grant from the W. K. Kellogg Foundation enabled establishment of the network; a grant of $1 million from the New York State Department of Health allowed expansion of a treatment site at I.S. 164 and the purchase of a new van; and a $150,000 grant from the Paula Vial Lampert Foundation provided funding for the original mobile van program. The College of Dental Medicine was grateful to the Alex Rodriguez Foundation's support of $250,000 for a new van to replace the original van, which wore out from use. The asthma

Acknowledgments

and immunization initiatives received additional grants from the Center
for Disease Control and Prevention, the New York State Department of
Health, Bank of America, and the Merck Foundation.

We were both surprised and delighted with the willingness of the chapter authors to step up to the plate and prepare their stories. We are deeply grateful to the authors and coauthors who took the time from their extremely busy schedules to write their stories. They are: David Albert, Yisel Alonzo, Mario Drummonds, Sally E. Findley, Laura Frye, Sandra Harris, Matilde Irigoyen, Kathleen Klink, Harris K. (Ken) Lampert, Anita Lee, María Lizardo, Stephen Marshall, Rosa Madera-Reese, Jacqueline Martínez, James McIntosh, Miriam Mejía, Dennis Mitchell, Benjamin Ortiz, Martin Ovalles, Moisés Pérez, Cheryl Ragonesi, Daniel F. Seidman, Martha Sánchez, Susan Sturm, and Gloria Thomas. We recognize the contributions of Walid Michelen in helping us prepare this book. His interview and written account helped form the context for various chapters. While he served as vice president for community affairs at the New York Presbyterian Hospital and co-chair of the Health Promotion/Disease Prevention Working Group, he was always a champion for the Northern Manhattan Community Voices Collaborative. Dr. Edward Healton, another champion of the NMCVC, often smoothed our pathway in his then role as Columbia's Associate Dean for the Harlem Hospital affiliation. We are grateful to Jennifer Stark for her superb research and editorial assistance on the final chapter of the book and to Shirley Torho for reference work.

We would be remiss if we did not acknowledge the vitality of the northern Manhattan community and its leadership who helped nurture the Northern Manhattan Community Voices Collaborative. Several of the community leaders are authors or coauthors of chapters and they are acknowledged above. In addition, many individuals are highlighted in the various stories in the book. We express our deepest respect, admiration, and gratitude for their contributions. Without them, these past ten years would not have been possible and we would not have had this story to tell. Of all of our community collaborators, Thelma C. Davidson Adair deserves special mention. She has been a guiding light for us in the Harlem community and was always available to lend a helping hand whenever we hit roadblocks.

Finally, a special acknowledgment to Shelley Lopez, who assisted the writing team in so many ways by taking care of details (including the food!) that made our meetings to prepare the book productive and eased our communications with the various partners.

Mobilizing the Community for Better Health

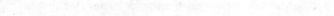

Part I
Beginnings

This part provides the background necessary to understand the origins of the Northern Manhattan Community Voices Collaborative (NMCVC). It includes a description of the community in which the collaborative was created, the partnership that developed, and the structure, operation, and management of the collaborative.

Introduction

The Northern Manhattan Community
Voices Collaborative

ALLAN J. FORMICOLA and LOURDES HERNÁNDEZ-CORDERO

The Great Society legislation of the 1960s started a social, economic, and medical transformation in America signaling to all that poor people and older people should have access to health care supported by government sponsored insurance. With the enactment of Medicaid and Medicare, particularly, many believed that such access would no longer be a privilege, but a right for everyone. However in the intervening years we have learned that the government and private system of health care has still left approximately 45 million Americans with no access to basic health care coverage, and that there are well over 108 million Americans with no dental insurance. America's unique and historical link between health care insurance coverage and some forms of employment is partly responsible for this gap.

However, while our spotty insurance coverage furnishes part of the explanation, it does not account for the whole picture of the health of our nation. In addition, even for many full-time employed Americans, there are large gaps in health status based on race, ethnicity, and income. Reports from the Institute of Medicine, such as *Unequal Treatment: Confronting Racial and Ethic Disparities in Health Care* (Smedley, Stith, and Kelson 2003), urge a keener sense of cultural awareness to improve the health of all Americans. Greater attention to poor health behaviors through prevention and better management of chronic disease can lead us to a higher quality of health while containing costs. These reforms to improve the health care system in the United States are now well known and their effectiveness well documented. As we completed this book in the fall of 2009, the nation was once again in the midst of actively considering reforms to the health care system that will cover all Americans and improve the quality of care. It is clear to us, however, that no matter how the debate turns out—the compromises that government will make to provide greater access to health and the systemic changes that the medical field puts into place to improve the quality of care—there will continue to be underserved population groups living in inner cities and rural areas that are marginalized in regard to health. These groups will continue to depend on a safety net of providers—some of them outside the formal health care system—to serve them.

The safety net, however, is ill defined, stretched thin, and difficult to access. While this book is not a cure-all, it deals with how northern Manhattan, an underserved low-income area, brought together a wide collaboration to shore up the safety net and make the health care system more responsive to local conditions. Solutions to health care system problems will be found at the national and state levels, but it is the changes that happen at the local level that can have a major impact on improving health. This book tells the story of how, through an academic–community partnership, a group of organizations went about making strategic changes to improve health care access and preventive care for its constituents.

In the late 1990s the W. K. Kellogg Foundation recognized that community-driven change has the potential to improve access and quality for the most vulnerable members of our society. In the call for proposals, the foundation recognized the importance of the safety net in providing basic care for underserved populations. In 1998 it launched a major $55 million initiative, Community Voices: Health Care for the Underserved, to form local partnerships to undertake grass-roots efforts to make the health care system better for their residents. The foundation selected thirteen sites from around the nation. At the same time as this book is published, a book describing the national Community Voices program will also be published by Jossey-Bass. Entitled *Community Voices: Health Matters*, the book has descriptions of all of the participating sites.

This book tells the story of one of the thirteen sites funded by the Kellogg Foundation, the Northern Manhattan Community Voices Collaborative (NMCVC). It describes the development of partnerships, the challenges faced by the collaborating entities, the processes put into place, and the outcomes, both successful and unsuccessful, between people in the institutions and community-based organizations striving to make northern Manhattan a healthier and better place to live.

For ten years, from 1998 to 2008, the NMCVC brought together leaders from institutions, churches, and community-based organizations to carry out a far-reaching plan to improve the general and oral health in the Washington Heights/Inwood and Harlem communities. With a high proportion of African Americans (in Harlem) and Latinos (in Washington Heights/Inwood), the socioeconomic markers and community health profile showed that both communities suffered from many of the problems typical of inner city residents.

Northern Manhattan has a population of approximately 400,000 people living in crowded neighborhoods and facing challenges related to poverty and the synergy of comorbidities of asthma, diabetes, and a host of other chronic illnesses. During the decade, managed care for the Medicaid population was being phased into the community, thus complicating many of the long-standing relationships that had built up between providers and community residents. There was considerable unrest in the community over health care issues. In general, the residents were suspicious of the large institutions in the community, which included Columbia University, Columbia University Medical Center, New York Presbyterian Hospital, and Harlem Hospital, because of past grievances about job opportunities, research studies without a lasting service component or translating the results into practice, and facility expansion plans in the neighborhoods.

Each of the communities has its own distinct character. Harlem is steeped in the African American culture, predicated partly on the fact that local churches are expected to provide important religious—as well as social, economic, and political—leadership to its residents. Washington Heights/Inwood, on the other hand, has served as a welcoming community to many waves of immigrants over the better part of the twentieth century. There have been successive changes in a variety of immigrant groups. Once largely an Irish and later an Eastern European Jewish enclave, today the community's makeup is largely Latino, the result of an influx of immigrants from the Dominican Republic beginning in the 1960s, and most recently of Central and South Americans beginning in the 1990s. This required lifestyle changes that were dramatic for both the receiving community and newcomers alike.

The Northern Manhattan Community Voices Collaborative believed that it could bring something different and worthwhile to the table within this social dynamic: a group of representative individuals from the institutions and the community committed to improving the overall health of the community while strengthening the safety net providers. This book brings out the manner in which the NMCVC worked and the results of its efforts. It describes and provides insight into the NMCVC itself, and its various achievements and struggles. We believed that it was necessary to write this book in order to put into perspective the massive effort that went into this collaboration.

In retrospect, the working symbiosis that resulted from the NMCVC between the local churches, community-based organizations (CBOs), and the large university and hospitals can be viewed as an important step in a détente between the lack of trust and differing viewpoints of community and institutional leaders. The churches and the CBOs had little trust in the large institutions and wanted health matters viewed in the context of social conditions. The institutions, on the other hand, were wary of inviting the community into their deliberations and viewed health matters pragmatically, that is, from the perspective of providing treatment for diseases, rather than through measures to promote health, prevent disease, and improve the social environment.

The tug between socioeconomic factors at play in the community and specific disease prevention interventions was often obvious throughout the life of the NMCVC. Nevertheless, by working together in the collaboration, a measure of trust was established between community and institutions over the years, even though major issues continue to separate them. Most important, though, is the fact that the collaborative demonstrated that solutions worked out on the grass-roots level between institution and community can lead to benefits for both. The lesson is clear: that open and frank dialogue brought about in a constructive environment can yield solutions to difficult problems for all involved.

One of the problems associated with large-scale community programs such as this one is how to design and implement evaluation procedures. The literature shows that most collaborative, community-wide programs struggle to assess the outcomes of their efforts, and the NMCVC is no exception. However, evaluation measures were built into the original collaborative model, and the Kellogg Foundation hired external evaluators to view the progress of each Community Voices site. While we draw upon this

information wherever possible, this book itself is our way to provide quali-
tative analysis of the challenges and accomplishments of the NMCVC.
Another important clarification about this type of project is that the Northern Manhattan Community Voices Collaborative was set up to respond to
service needs and not to be a classic research project, but as the reader will
note in the various chapters, research did come out of the project. For example, the outcomes of the asthma and immunization projects (chapters 4
and 5) and the SASA project (chapter 7) are reported. Many of the other
chapters report outcomes data; the principle we followed was that the
research findings were a *by-product of the service initiative* rather than
vice-versa.

The NMCVC addresses a major question: can urban research universities successfully collaborate with their surrounding communities? For that
collaboration to be effective, the NMCVC set forth to initiate four major
systems changes:

1. Enhance community-based primary care network services to include neighborhood-by-neighborhood health promotion and disease prevention efforts.
2. Extend outreach to increase enrollment in Medicaid and Child
   Health Plus.
3. Improve the provider network's capacity to offer targeted services
   for difficult-to-cover services, including dental and behavioral/
   mental health services.
4. Develop and implement an insurance product to enroll more of
   the uninsured.

These very ambitious goals were set out in 1998. The NMCVC mission
statement drafted at the inception of the project included the following:
"An ultimate goal is to create a northern Manhattan community that educates itself about health issues and secures needed health resources from
public authorities and private sources." In other words, the collaboration
intended to build the capacity of the community to deal with its health
problems.

Since the goal of building community capacity was a priority, the Northern Manhattan Community Voices Collaborative did not set out to be a research project, as mentioned earlier. However, throughout the years, principles of Community Based Participatory Research (CBPR) were used to

8
Beginnings

lead the examination of health issues and determine programmatic direction. Furthermore, CBPR strategies were used in the development of an agenda for the Health Promotion Working Group and for the background research leading to the White Paper on Mental Health.[1]

To build capacity from the onset, the collaborative sought to implement community mobilization strategies to engage partners from the community, local institutions, and government agencies. Community mobilization has its roots in political and social movements and has been documented extensively in the political science, sociology, and anthropology literatures (Vanecko 1969; Jackson 1978). With the increased attention that public health practitioners and researchers have given to the study of health disparities over the past fifteen years, community mobilization has emerged as an important strategy for facilitating change to address these disparities. In our work, we have relied on Freire's work on education for action, specifically his *Pedagogy of the Oppressed*. Freire's work proposes education and engagement as a means to leverage the social and political power of—using public health language—underserved populations. We expanded the interpretation of Freire's work to propose that through education and engagement health needs can be identified, innovative solutions proposed, and resources leveraged. Thus, we built on the resources available in the community and worked to build the capacity of the community to better itself in regard to health. Working though existing community-based organizations to plan and implement various initiatives and building the human resources by the education of community-health workers, for example, are classic ways to involve the community in initiatives.

In carrying out its mission, the NMCVC emphasized the notion that pilot projects and programs around the systems changes it envisioned needed to identify the way in which they would be institutionalized and sustained. In keeping with Freire's work, this could be accomplished only by significant and well-informed engagement of community partners, not simply through academic or institutional leadership. The collaborative was limited by its intention to begin only those projects and programs that could be institutionalized after the grant funds ended. As readers will note, some of the initiatives were successfully institutionalized while others were not.

While this method of engagement permeated the ten years of the collaborative work postfunding, we acknowledge that there was limited time available for dialogue between the community and the institutions prior to funding (in preparing and submitting the Kellogg grant proposal). Although the success of a community-based program can be tied to the manner in which the project was planned among the partners, the NMCVC needed to follow the goals and objectives set out in the grant as it was designed by the Kellogg Foundation and its team of experts. The three partners of the NMCVC—Columbia University Medical Center (College of Dental Medicine), Alianza Dominicana, and Harlem Hospital (Dental Service)—had little time to do more than touch base with many important constituents during the planning phase; however, in addition to these three organizations, many others endorsed the collaboration and participated in the collaborative. The three partners had intimate knowledge about each of the constituencies that would be involved, that is, the university/hospitals and the communities of Harlem and Washington Heights/Inwood. We further recognized that once funded, all the activities of the NMCVC needed to be widely collaborative and, over the life span of the NMCVC, more than thirty-five community-based organizations and institutions became involved in the collaborative endeavors.

The Kellogg Foundation initially funded the thirteen Community Voices sites as "Learning Laboratories." Each would share its successes and failures, best practices would be determined, and each would receive five years of funding as a demonstration site. The foundation also provided another four years of follow-up support for eight of the thirteen sites—extra funding to carry out policy work that would be needed to maintain initiatives undertaken in the first five years. The NMCVC was one of the sites that received an initial five-year grant and a four-year follow-up grant to advocate for policy to sustain the initiatives. Thus, the NMCVC has had the rare opportunity to have almost ten years of experience working with a community in which providers strain to meet the needs of residents who often are suspicious of the motives of the institutions.

As is the case with Community Voices, this book itself represents a collaborative effort. The core editorial team gave the book its initial shape—a shape that changed as the chapters were written. From the beginning, we felt that each NMCVC project had a story that was unique and needed to be told in its own way. The chapter authors are the people who were in the thick of things: staff members of the partner institutions and community-based organizations. They aimed to tell the story in their own style, and they include relevant bumps in the road, setbacks, and unmet goals; similarly, they reveal strokes of fortune and events or conditions that made the process easier and more successful. We directed the authors to prepare their chapters as engaging stories and to limit their references to only five or six. The resulting chapters show that the NMCVC attracted a variety of different people, and as unique individuals each decided the best way to tell their story. In addition, the literature supporting some of the initiatives is extensively quoted in some of the chapters (chapters 3, 4, 5, 7, and 10), while other chapters are written in a more narrative style without extensive supporting literature or theoretical framework. Wherever possible in the latter, a list of suggested additional references on selected topics that may be of interest to some readers follows the chapter references.

To gain further insight into the environment in which the NMCVC began its work, we interviewed a variety of individuals, from members of community-based organizations to community residents, and from key staff of the NMCVC to students. The interviews were conducted in two ways: written or oral responses to a set of questions posed to individuals and/or taped interviews. The taped interviews provided an opportunity for the interviewees to expand on their answers. In all, eighteen interviews were held over a period of approximately one year. Even though most of these interviews were conducted ten years after the initiation of the Community Voices program in New York, their recollections were astonishingly vivid and fresh. Those interviewed were able to reflect back on the collaboration as well as to assess accomplishments. Similar to the diversity of the community and the institutions in which the NMCVC was set, those interviewed had a diverse set of answers to the questions posed. Their answers enliven the chapters. In addition, archival materials (annual reports, meeting minutes, and internal documents) were utilized to provide context and factual evidence.

Each chapter in this book shows how the NMCVC went about the challenges in meeting the goals of the four systems changes it envisioned in its Kellogg grant: health promotion, outreach, provision of targeted services, and insurance for the underserved. The book articulates many specific, concrete lessons learned in the process and places them in the context of how the Columbia University Medical Center worked with its surrounding community, and vice versa, to improve the health safety net in northern Manhattan.

The book is divided into five parts. The first part—this introduction and chapters 1 and 2—provides background information on the Kellogg Foundation's Community Voices initiative and a description of the partners who formed the NMCVC and the management and operation of the collaborative. The second (chapters 3–6), third (chapters 7–10), and fourth parts (chapters 11–13) tell the stories behind the specific projects designed to bring about the systems changes funded by the Kellogg Foundation and the other funders that the collaborative was able to attract. The final section (chapters 14 and 15) analyzes the accomplishments and challenges of the NMCVC, systems changes, and the lessons learned that can be applied to the national scene.

Thus, chapter 1 explains who the partners are and how they came together as the NMCVC, while chapter 2 specifically deals with the structure, operation, and management of the NMCVC.

Chapter 3 describes how and why community-health workers became a key strategy to implement many of the collaborative's initiatives, as well as the development of Alianza Dominicana, a community-based organization and NMCVC partner, as a major influence in improving northern Manhattan. Next covered are health promotion programs to improve asthma control in children (chapter 4), increase the immunization rate (chapter 5), and reduce tobacco use in the community (chapter 6). Chapters 5 and 6 were developed through extensive dialogue with the community and with a keen eye to sustainability. The tobacco initiative (chapter 6) grew out of a partnership between the Kellogg Foundation and the American Legacy Foundation to counteract tobacco companies' targeted advertisement to youngsters, especially in low-income communities.

Chapter 7 shows that an intervention at the level of the emergency room (department) can move habitual users into primary care. Chapter 8 describes the Health Information Tool for Empowerment, a partnership that improves the capacity of community-based agencies to find care for clients using the Internet. Health depends on good nutrition and exercise; chapter 9 describes a pilot project called Healthy Choices between the school system and the NMCVC, which educated parents and children to improve dietary intake and increase physical activity. The hard-to-cover services in most underserved communities are dental and mental health care. Chapters 10 and 11, respectively, tell the story of the development of a far-reaching dental network called Community DentCare and how a mental health report set the stage to improve mental health initiatives in the communities. Chapter 12 describes the saga of setting up and operating the Thelma Adair Medical/Dental Center, a primary care health facility in central Harlem. While the NMCVC was unsuccessful in developing a new insurance product for uninsured, chapter 13 describes lessons learned in the process of developing such a plan and in a way foretells some of the same financial issues facing the nation as it tries to devise ways to provide coverage for all of the population.

The penultimate chapter, chapter 14 sums up and analyzes the systems changes and challenges, successes and failures, of the NMCVC; the final chapter, chapter 15 proposes that the lessons learned could be scaled up to the larger national picture. In this chapter the book returns to the broader question of how an institution and community collaboration can bring about a much needed reform to improve the health of society, especially for those living in low-income communities. We suggest a way the academic health schools and centers and their respective communities can develop, through collaboration and the lessons learned in the NMCVC, a national prevention program.

The overarching principle that emerged from the relationships that developed between the safety net providers, faculty and health providers, and the community was that we learned from each other. Community members came to the table with different experiences from those of the providers and faculty, and vice versa. By mixing them together in a structure that encouraged listening, the collaboration was able to create a cooperative working climate that often accomplished more than had been expected. Those who subscribe to John Dewey's and the aforementioned Paulo Freire's philosophies of education have long advocated active education of this type. Each individual and the community at large benefited from the interaction. The final chapter applies this principle to scaling up the program nationally. In the epilogue, we describe how the NMCVC became embedded into the fiber of the institutions and the community through the progress of the individuals who learned by working in the initiative. While the NMCVC as an entity no longer exists, it lives on through these individuals and through improved relationships between the safety net providers and the community.

In an interview Karina Feliz, program supervisor at Alianza Dominicana, the largest social services organization for Dominicans in the country and NMCVC partner, expressed the legacy by defining the collaboration: "it's basically what the name is, Community Voices, reaching out to the community, educating the community, empowering the community." Karina became one of the NMCVC's community scholars and through that scholarship completed her master's degree in public health. Essentially, this is what we hoped to create: a structure that would help the community deal with the problems it faced. It is the desire to contribute to the national dialog about improving the health of underserved communities, by disseminating the story of these successes and failures, that drove us to write this book.

Note

1. For an in-depth examination of CBPR principles and case studies, we recommend the work of Meredith Minkler and Nina Wallerstein.

References

Institute for the Future (2003). *Health & health care 2010: The forecast, the challenge.* San Francisco: Jossey-Bass.

Jackson, Pamela I. (1978). Community control, community mobilization, and community political structure in 57 U.S. cities. *Sociological Quarterly* 19, no. 4: 577.

Minkler, M., and N. Wallerstein (eds.) (2008). *Community-based participatory research for health: From process to outcomes.* 2nd edition. San Francisco: Jossey-Bass.

Smedley, B., A. Stith, and A. Kelson, A. (eds.). (2003). *Unequal treatment: Confronting racial and ethnic disparities in health care.* Institute of Medicine. Washington, D.C.: National Academies Press.

Vanecko, James J. (1969). Community mobilization and institutional change: The influence of the community action program in large cities. *Social Science Quarterly* 50, no. 3: 609.

W. K. Kellogg Foundation (2002). *More than a market: Making sense of health care systems. Lessons from Community Voices: Health care for the underserved.* Battle Creek, Mich.: W. K. Kellogg Foundation. http://www.communityvoices.org.

[1]

Creating the Collaborative Foundation

ALLAN J. FORMICOLA, MOISÉS PÉREZ, and JAMES MCINTOSH

Relationships are primary and everything else is secondary.

—Ron David

This book is about accomplishments of an unusual and powerful collaboration that fueled a number of important initiatives to improve the health of the people living in northern Manhattan. While recording these accomplishments by themselves is important, so is documenting the way they came about. We believe that the structure we put into place was partly responsible for the success of the effort, especially in the pivotal first few years when ideas moved to specific plans and then to action. Equally important, however, is the role of the people who became involved with the NMCVC, the leaders who actually believed in the mission and built the engine that kept moving us forward. In the book *Good to Great*, Jim Collins (2001:41) pointed out the importance of getting the "right people on the bus"; once this is accomplished the company's executive can "figure out how to take it [the company] someplace great."

In this chapter, you will learn about the early steps we took in getting the right people on the bus in order to get the grant, laying the foundation for the right organizational structure, and shaping the two guiding principles (see page 22) of the collaborative that set everything else in motion.

First Steps: The Three Partners

Partnerships come together because they can achieve something that each partner cannot achieve individually. This was the case with the partnership that arose to respond to the W. K. Kellogg Foundation's Call for Proposals for its major national initiative, Community Voices: Health Care for the Underserved. From the very beginning, we knew that there would be intense competition to obtain a Community Voices grant and that the intention of the foundation was to build local efforts that had the potential and leadership to help shore up the fragile safety net providers in the United States. We had previously worked together on community issues and decided that a partnership between us would be very attractive in obtaining a grant.

One of us represented a highly respected research university, Columbia University; another, a major safety net hospital, Harlem Hospital; and the third, an active community-based organization, Alianza Dominicana. All three of us were located in northern Manhattan where over 400,000 mainly low-income individuals lived and struggled with obtaining health care. During his deanship of the College of Dental Medicine of Columbia University, Allan Formicola had extensive working relations with Harlem Hospital and especially with James McIntosh, the director of the Dental Service. We developed a successful program enrolling dental residents of Harlem Hospital into specialty programs at the Columbia College of Dental Medicine (Formicola et al. 2003). Moisés Pérez, chief executive officer of Alianza, worked closely with Formicola and McIntosh in the planning and development of the Community DentCare network, an extensive outreach project of the dental college that aimed to bring dental care to children in convenient locations in the public schools and in neighborhoods (Formicola et al. 1999). (In fact, the newly forming Kellogg-funded partnership was to play a future role in the DentCare program, as told in chapter 11.) McIntosh and Formicola had also worked closely together in garnishing the necessary resources to build the dental service at Harlem Hospital from primarily one that took care of acute dental problems such as extractions to one that provided extensive restorative care as well as acute care.

All three of us were risk takers and not afraid to take on challenges. We recognized that collaboration leads to better outcomes than trying to solve problems alone. When we sat down to prepare the application for the W. K. Kellogg Foundation initiative, it was the trust that had built up among us that permitted us to create one of the thirteen approved Kellogg Community Voices projects in the United States. The structure we created to operate our proposal was called the Northern Manhattan Community Voices Collaborative. We chose the name deliberately to emphasize the collaborative aspect of the initiative.

Backdrop: A Complex Community

Northern Manhattan was—and still is—a dynamic and complex environment. It would be necessary for multiple individuals throughout the community's institutions to become knowledgeable about the grant proposal and give approval for submitting it. At the time of submission, the institutional and community environment had formidable challenges to overcome for the partners to submit a cooperative application. There was considerable mistrust between the northern Manhattan community and the university and its medical center.

As detailed in table 1.1, residents in Washington Heights and Inwood, the most northern reaches of Manhattan, are mainly Hispanic, and most are recent immigrants from the Dominican Republic. Harlem is largely an African American community that had experienced much poverty over the last half of the twentieth century. Both communities viewed Presbyterian Hospital (now known as New York Presbyterian Hospital), the major teaching hospital affiliated with Columbia's health science schools, as well as Columbia University as mainly interested in the community from a research perspective. The community's perspective about the institutions is that they had experienced too many university projects that involved research with little to no long-term benefit to the community. Although Presbyterian Hospital was the only remaining hospital in this northern portion of Manhattan and had built off-site ambulatory facilities in northern Manhattan in addition to a small community hospital, the sheer size of the institution was intimidating.

The hospital had only recently appointed a high-level physician, Dr. Walid Michelen, with responsibilities to improve relations with the surrounding community. Dr. Michelen became a strong advocate and working member of the NMCVC. The administration for the health sciences schools (Schools of Medicine, Dentistry, Public Health, and Nursing) had established an office of government and community affairs in the

TABLE 1.1

Demographic, Socioeconomic, and Health Characteristics
of Northern Manhattan, 2000

	WASHINGTON HEIGHTS/INWOOD	HARLEM	NORTHERN MANHATTAN
Total Population	208,414	218,833	427,247
Latino	74%	30%	52%
African American	13%	56%	33%
Foreign born	51%	20%	32%
Population <5 years old	18,664	12,133	30,797
Median family income, 1999	$28,451	$24,295	$26,184
Households with income < poverty level	31%	37%	34%

Source: 2000 population and socioeconomic statistics from the U.S. Census; health data from the New York City DOHMH Community Survey 2004.

1980s. The community affairs officer, Ivy Fairchild, also a Dominican and daughter of Washington Heights, recognized that the Community Voices initiative had the potential of improving relations with the surrounding communities and with Harlem Hospital, for which the College of Physicians and Surgeons and the College of Dental Medicine provided the professional staff.

The vision for the Northern Manhattan Community Voices Collaborative was the instrument that galvanized all to work together. The disease levels in the community exceeded those of many other communities in New York City and in the nation. In fact, a study by two Harlem Hospital doctors concluded that a Harlem man's chances of living past the age of forty were less than those of the average male resident of Bangladesh—one of the poorest countries in the world (McCord and Freeman 1990). Harlem also fared poorly for most measures of health. The mission for the collaboration therefore became to promote systems change to focus on disease prevention and create a system shift toward wellness in health care delivery.

The idea was to build community-wide interventions by developing working relations with community-based organizations and leaders within the safety net health institutions in northern Manhattan. Such a shift had been promoted by many leaders in the medical field beginning in the 1970s, but making it happen has proven difficult, especially in communities where taking care of acute needs strains the safety net providers. Could the NMCVC help to promote such a systems shift in northern Manhattan? The proposal to Kellogg was both broad in concept and specific in the manner in which the collaborative would organize the local initiative to carry out this vision. We were convinced that we could build cooperative relations with the various institutions and community organizations to institute transformation in the health care system in northern Manhattan.

Each in our own way had intimate knowledge of our community and constituents. McIntosh, an African American dentist, lived in Harlem and had a private dental practice, served as chief of the Dental Service at Harlem Hospital, and held longtime leadership positions in the local health care institutions. Pérez, a Dominican, had built Alianza Dominicana as a social organization that viewed health from a holistic perspective based on improving the overall environment of the community. Pérez's links to the medical center were with the cofounder of the organization he directed, Rafael Lantigua, a Dominican physician who served on the medical school's faculty. Formicola held an influential position as dean of the dental college for more than fifteen years and established the Community DentCare plan, which reached out into the public schools and neighborhoods. He served on many university and hospital committees and understood the culture within the university and the medical center. All three of us understood that the specific objectives for the NMCVC had to be far reaching while dealing with grass-roots problems that people faced.

Our Four Objectives

From our individual and collective knowledge, we set up four specific objectives for the NMCVC. We understood that there were many residents in the community who were eligible for health care coverage under Medicaid but either feared to sign up for it or did not understand the process to obtain coverage; therefore, the first objective involved increasing the enrollment of the residents into existing insurance programs. We realized that there were many individuals living in the community who, for example, worked in small businesses and had no insurance plans in which they were eligible, so the second objective was to explore how to obtain coverage for this group. There was a lack of prevention programs in the community, and thus the third objective became to promote health education and disease prevention measures, especially for diseases such as diabetes and asthma, which were at epidemic proportions in northern Manhattan. And, finally, we realized that access to dental and mental health care were lacking—as they are in the general population for a variety of reasons—and that these hard-to-cover services needed a specific targeted effort. Once the NMCVC was organized around these four objectives, we then created a structure consisting of an executive group, a large steering committee and four working groups, each one of which was responsible for one of the objectives. (The story of creating the structure is told in greater detail in chapter 2.)

Getting the Grant

The competition for the grants was intense. More than eighty proposals were submitted to the foundation. There were five proposals from New York City alone, including the NMCVC's. We came through Kellogg's thorough proposal review successfully because we had good support throughout the university, the hospital, and the community for the proposal. At the site visit many leaders spoke up for the proposal and indicated that they wished to be part of it. The foundation awarded the NMCVC with one of its largest five-year grants, $4.5 million. Of the thirteen sites awarded grants, NMCVC was the only one where dentistry was in the leadership position and the only grant awarded in the Northeast. The foundation referred to the sites as "learning laboratories" since the lessons learned from each were expected to inform the national dialog on how to improve the health care system for underserved populations.

While we did not know how we would achieve this last goal at the time of the writing of the grant, it became apparent—as we progressed through annual meetings, published papers, and reports, and as we heard from visitors to our site—that many learned from our examples. We did not set out to write this book; however, the publication of it is another way to share our experience. The Kellogg Foundation too has understood the need to disseminate the lessons learned and has funded the Morehouse School of Medicine with grants to disseminate lessons learned.

Dividing up the budget is often the stumbling block for successful collaboration. And the discussion on the budget was difficult, as would be expected. However, the budget discussions actually flowed from the collaborative's objectives rather than from the idea of dividing up the spoils in a political way. Alianza received a five-year budget of $1.5 million to undertake increasing the enrollment of the residents into Medicaid and Child Health Plus and to provide leadership on infusing promotoras (community health workers) into the work of partner organizations and institutions. The Community Premier Plus, the Medicaid Managed Care Company of three safety net hospitals (New York Presbyterian, Harlem, and North General), received $650,000 to develop insurance plans for those ineligible for existing insurance, and the remainder ($2.4 million) went to the dental college to administer the grant and take on planning and pilot testing the health promotion/disease prevention and mental/dental health objectives. Some of these latter funds were provided to the School of Public Health for a Community Voices scholars program. We understood that the NMCVC had an educational role to play and that it could provide a setting for the education of public health students and other health science students.

The Executive Directors

With the grant approved in 1998, the first task was to fill the crucial position of full-time executive director. We needed someone who could put together a team that could manage the overall direction of the NMCVC as well as the details of each of its subprojects, to turn the written plan into reality. Over the course of the grant, three extremely capable people filled this post.

The executive committee conducted an extensive search for the first director and was fortunate to recruit Sandra Harris. Harris was born in the Dominican Republic and raised in Washington Heights. Her college major was psychology and individual and group counseling, perfect for what she would end up doing in her career. She earned her college degree while working first as a community assistant and later as the district office director for New York State Senator Franz Leichter. Then, while working at Alianza Dominicana on mental illness prevention and teen pregnancy prevention programs, she continued on to earn a MSW degree at Hunter College. Both positions allowed her to develop relationships with key stakeholders in the nonprofit sector as well as with surrounding institutions.

Harris had the administrative skill set and personality to manage this broad collaboration. She remained as executive director through the first five-year grant and into the first year of the subsequent four-year grant. A large degree of the success of the effort goes to Harris because not only did she have the ability to manage the organization for action, she also had long-standing relationships with many of the community partners we convened. She brought with her the respect and trust that takes years to build and that can make or break an initiative. Harris stayed long enough to have continuity in the work of the collaborative toward its goals.

Jacqueline Martínez succeeded Harris in 2003 as executive director. Harris had hired Martínez earlier to staff one of the working groups, and she too had been raised in the community. Martínez earned a bachelor of science degree from Cornell majoring in human development and then completed a master's degree in public health from Columbia. Martínez had many of the same skill sets that Harris had. Prior to joining Community Voices, Martínez had completed a major paper for a Kaiser Family Foundation project on racial and ethnic disparities in diagnosis and treatment in the U.S. health care system. Both Harris and Martínez were deeply committed to improving the community, so the NMCVC was fortunate to have two excellent, highly intelligent, and deeply committed executive directors for the better part of its nine-year history.

As we came to the end of the effort, we were again fortunate to have a ready team in place to take over. Lourdes Hernández-Cordero, a Puerto Rican native and Community Voices scholar who prepared the Mental Health Report for Community Voices (see chapter 12), earned a doctoral degree in public health and was an assistant professor in the School of Public Health when she took over as the final executive director in the tenth year of the project. She was assisted by Yisel Alonzo. Alonzo had joined the effort earlier, working on developing an electronic directory for health services (see chapter 8) and a diet and nutrition program (see chapter 10). One of the reasons why the NMCVC has been successful is the quality of these individuals and the fact that they were able to gain experience in the organization or with one of the founding members prior to assuming leadership roles. In addition, these individuals have become the doers for getting this book written and have contributed chapters as well as overall direction.

Shortly after the grants were awarded, the foundation held its first annual meeting, in Stowe, Vermont. Attending for the NMCVC were Formicola,

Pérez, Walid Michelen (Presbyterian Hospital), Harris, and Marshall England, a community organizer in Harlem who served on Harlem Hospital's Community Board. McIntosh thought it best to send England to this meeting rather than himself as he realized that England was a powerful force in Harlem and wanted him to become well steeped in the collaborative. This meeting cemented the relationships between these individuals, and over the next five years they were able to bring the NMCVC into a lively organization that accomplished much. (Unfortunately, Marshall England died suddenly around the third year of the collaboration. He was a wonderful community leader who had the capability of sizing up people and deciding whether they were truly committed to the community or not.)

One of the outstanding talks at the Stowe meeting that reflected England's philosophy was by a young physician, Ron David, who began his remarks with the following notion: "relationships are primary and everything else is secondary." In retrospect, these eight words are the ones that describe how the NMCVC unfolded. When the relationships were right, the collaboration accomplished much; when they were not, vice versa. Fortunately, they were right most of the time.

Two Guiding Operational Principles

We understood that for the collaborative to be successful it would have to be guided by two operational principles. We knew at some point that the NMCVC would go out of existence, so the first was that the collaborative should only deal in *stimulating* change through pilot projects or studies that had identified institutions or organizations that could institutionalize the effort. This recognized that the existing institutions and community-based organizations could develop the capacity to adopt the various projects, and that the main idea behind Community Voices was to build the capacity in the community rather than to create a large new infrastructure that could not maintain itself. The second principle was that the collaborative would have to become known in the institutions and the community in order to get its goals and objectives achieved, but that the credit for the success of its individual initiatives would accrue to others. In other words, the NMCVC could have no ego but instead must be satisfied to know that it seeded efforts to improve the health safety net in northern Manhattan.

These guiding principles helped plant and nourish many successful initiatives that have sustained themselves. In evaluating the outcome of the NMCVC "learning laboratory," the two principles—along with the guiding light about relationships being primary—are the most important lessons that have emerged out of the past ten years. Many of the individuals who began with the project in one capacity or another have moved onto successful positions enhancing their new organizations' capacity. The NMCVC legacy then is in demonstrating that institutions and community can overcome mistrust and come together to create transformational change— change that can lead to creating much needed new service programs building upon the strengths and resources of those who invest themselves in the community. In chapters 3–13, those individuals who were instrumental in bringing about the changes tell the stories that have improved the capacity of the community and the capacity of the institutional providers to gain a new understanding of their surrounding community.

Several big-picture outcomes came about over the life of the NMCVC. First, it was one of only eight of the original thirteen sites to receive a four-year continuation grant of $1 million after the initial five-year period. Second, the work of the collaborative attracted $45 million of other funding because others believed that its mission and way of operating were important. Third, the collaborative spawned new approaches to improving the health of the community. In reflecting back, Walid Michelen, now the chief of staff for Lincoln Medical and Mental Health Center, recently said, "There were major successes but some failures in the execution. Nevertheless, the successes greatly overshadowed the failures."

References

Collins, J. (2001). *Good to great: Why some companies make the leap . . . and others don't*. New York: HarperCollins.

David, R. (1998). Policy challenges and opportunities for the future: Impact on services for the underserved. *Proceedings of Networking Meeting, Community Voices Series*. W. K. Kellogg Foundation, August.

Formicola, A., J. Klyvert, A. McIntosh, M. Thompson, M. Davis, and T. Cangialosi (2003). Creating an environment for diversity in dental schools: One school's approach. *Journal of Dental Education* 676: 491–99.

Formicola, A., J. McIntosh, S. Marshall, D. Albert, D. Mitchell-Lewis, G. Zabos, and R. Garfield (1999). Population-based primary care and dental education: A new role for dental schools. *Journal of Dental Education* 63: 331–38.

McCord, C., and H. P. Freeman (1990) Excess mortality in Harlem of Harlem Hospital. *New England Journal of Medicine* 322, no. 3: 173–77. http://content.nejm.org/cgi/content/abstract/322/3/173.

2

The Collaborative Structure and the Challenges We Faced

SANDRA HARRIS

The devil is in the details.

—Variant of the proverb

There is an old saying: "Be careful what you wish for—you might get it." With the awarding of the Kellogg grant, we now needed to deliver on its goals and objectives. The structure we presented in the grant application had to come alive and manage this broad collaborative. Could that happen and would it work?

In chapter 1, the story of the three founding partners and the evolution of the two underlying principles of the Northern Manhattan Community Voices Collaborative was told. This chapter continues the story. We describe the organizational structure of the collaborative and discuss the challenges of working in a collaborative, including the challenges we faced in managing the complex goals of the NMCVC. Equally important, we introduce the key individuals who charted the way to move forward in transforming the ideas from paper to reality—the people we put on the bus to make this effort successful.

Three Bodies

The overall structure of the organization was designed to include three bodies: an administrative committee, the steering committee, and the

working groups. The administrative committee included the three founding partners from the sponsoring organizations, Allan J. Formicola (Columbia), Moisés Pérez (Alianza), and James McIntosh (Harlem Hospital),
and the executive director. The administrative committee eventually became an executive committee and was designed to assess overall progress
and set the direction for other groups. The steering committee was a much
larger group consisting of thirteen members broadly representing all the
elements of the collaboration. An official of the State Department of Health
also sat in on the meetings. The third body consisted of four working
groups assigned to develop and implement the four objectives of the project and another group to work on internal evaluation.

Could this structure actually lead to changing systems? Could it work?
The outcomes of the NMCVC include many accomplishments so the answer to the question is yes, it did work; it did stimulate change. But why
did this structure work and how did it work? What made it successful?

Two of the fundamental keys to our success were that many of the people who formed the collaborative already had a track record of working together and that each had the same vision to see the health of the northern
Manhattan community improved through new community-based strategies. The organizational partners represented on the steering committee
were able to move their organizations in the directions that were agreed
upon by the working groups. The working groups brought in additional
individuals—those at the grass-roots level who had the knowledge and experience to design initiatives that had a realistic chance of taking hold in
their institutions and organizations. The institutions and the community
were ready for this initiative, and that is probably another reason why the
collaborative worked. Walid Michelen, who had been chief medical officer
for the New York City Health and Hospitals Corporation and became cochair of one of the working groups, voices his motivation: "I wanted a
change from working on broad issues that had an impact on the city's
health policies and the delivery of quality services in all the boroughs. I
wanted to focus on one or two neighborhoods; to work more 'on the ground,'
where I could see the results of my work more directly; to not have to deal
with too much politics (you always have to deal with politics!); to focus less
on setting policy and dealing with immense institutions and more on improving the health of a defined population."

The Steering Committee

Once the leadership was in place, our next step was to activate the steering committee. The steering committee was given the responsibility for oversight of all NMCVC activities. Over the first five years of the NMCVC, the steering committee was very active and met regularly. It actually steered our overall initiatives!

The steering committee included many high-level individuals who had the clout to make sure that projects that touched their institutions or organizations moved ahead. The list of members was impressive (see table 2.1). It is very difficult for a large committee to steer a large community effort—and yet eventually we added even more individuals. What was important about the steering committee is that it met consistently during the critical first years of the initiative, received reports from the working groups, and discussed the initiatives that were to be taken. In essence, the initiatives brought to the committee had been well thought out by the working groups. Because the steering committee was thoroughly informed of the specific initiatives of the NMCVC, members could open the necessary doors in their sphere of influence to help the working groups make progress.

What set this steering committee apart from most others of this type was that the members were clear on the goals and objectives set forth by the collaborative. Thus, when new program initiatives and activities were brought to the table, the first question was: how does this move our overall mission forward? Working group chairs (or the executive director) had to present new program ideas and be prepared to discuss in detail how the project would contribute to the sustainability of improved health care outcomes. In addition, members of the steering committee were at the front line of their respective organizations, and this allowed them to relate to the issues addressed by the collaborative and to contribute in tangible ways. Members volunteered to review grant applications, to meet prospective funders, and to facilitate meetings and conferences on behalf of the collaborative.

Keeping the steering committee engaged in the development of the collaborative was key and required strong administrative oversight. For example, dates for meetings were submitted two to three months in advance to ensure maximum attendance and also to send the message to our members that their participation was critical to move our agenda. Indeed, the feedback obtained during our meetings proved to be critical and always

TABLE 2.1

The Steering Committee and Other Partners

ORIGINAL STEERING COMMITTEE, REPRESENTING SAFETY NET PROVIDERS AND
COMMUNITY/CHURCH ORGANIZATIONS IN NORTHERN MANHATTAN

Columbia University, College of Dental Medicine
Alianza Dominicana, Inc.
Harlem Hospital Dental Service
Ambulatory Care Network of the New York Presbyterian Hospital
Associates in Internal Medicine Group Practice (AIM)
Columbia University, College of Physicians and Surgeons
Columbia University, School of Public Heath
Community Premier Plus (A Managed Care Insurance Company)
Harlem Congregations for Community Improvement
Harlem Hospital Administration
Harlem Hospital Community Advisory Board
Presbyterian Hospital (now New York Presbyterian Hospital)
Renaissance Health Care Network

ADDITIONAL ORGANIZATIONS THAT JOINED THE COLLABORATION OVER THE ACTIVE YEARS
OF THE NMCVC AS THEY BECAME ENGAGED IN THE WORK

Abyssinian Baptist Church
Children's Aid Society
Children's Defense Fund
Columbia University School of Nursing
Community Health Worker Network of New York City
Community Impact
Community League of West 159th Street
Community Life Center
Council Health Center
Harlem Health Promotion Center
Inwood Community Services, Inc.
Isabella
National Alliance on Mental Illness (Harlem Chapter)
National Alliance on Mental Illness (New York City Metro Chapter)
New York City Department of Health and Mental Hygiene
New York State Department of Health
New York State Psychiatric Institute
Northern Manhattan Coalition for Immigrant Rights
Northern Manhattan Improvement Corporation
North General Hospital
Rheedlen Center (now known as the Ryan Center)
The Valley
West Harlem Environmental Action (WE ACT)

---

moved us to further work on behalf of the collaborative. Annual reports were never mailed—they were distributed at the meetings, with presentations from working groups and community partners highlighting the issues noted in the report.

Two sets of minutes of the steering committee place in perspective the progress of the collaborative. The minutes of a 1999 meeting show that toward the end of the first year of the project, momentum was building for the collaborative. The minutes noted that "we are moving from ideas and notions to actual projects and initiatives," and that the collaborative had submitted a grant to the state of New York to facilitate enrollment for Medicaid eligible residents. (This grant for $500,000 was subsequently approved.) Reports from the various working groups, for example, the Outreach and Enrollment group, indicated that four organizations (Children's Aid Society, School of Public Health, Children's Defense Fund, and Alianza Dominicana) began their first training of fifteen individuals as outreach workers. It was further noted that 446 individuals had been enrolled in Medicaid or Child Health Plus. Similar progress was noted from the other working groups.

A second set of minutes, of a meeting held at the end of the fourth year of the project, shows the enormous reach of the NMCVC. The minutes report the robust leveraging of the original grant funds: a total of an additional $45,560,000 was raised from a variety of other funders, a tenfold increase of the original $4.5 million grant. Additionally, members of the steering committee learned about the accomplishments of the various working groups and received a list of the twelve events that the NMCVC held in May 2002. These events ranged from organizing efforts for the tobacco cessation initiative, to immunization efforts, to an asthma media campaign and a community network subcommittee meeting. The steering committee meeting minutes demonstrate that in just four years this unwieldy collaborative had become a hub of important activities leading to change.

The Working Groups

The success of the NMCVC should largely be attributed to the working groups. It was the working groups that took on the various tasks necessary to achieve the goals and objectives set forth by the collaborative. The leadership of the working groups was instrumental in crystallizing the huge tasks ahead for the members. Each working group had cochairs who brought a wealth of expertise in their respective areas and had an established track record in brokering partner relationships in their field. The cochairs were individuals who had a keen understanding of the community and were committed to forging real changes in the areas that they led. The general membership of the working group comprised frontline staff at local organizations and the hospital. They brought the voices of the people they served on a daily basis. The cochairs turned to them when planning interventions, educational programs, and trainings.

Part of what made the working groups so dynamic was that we made sure that the membership was equally represented by academia and community-based organizations. The working groups gave both an opportunity to exchange ideas and learn from each other. (This posed a huge challenge for me as the executive director: I had to balance the need to make sure that they benefited from each other's strengths while being vigilant about one group not overpowering the other.)

There were four groups working in specific areas to improve the health of the community: (1) Outreach and Enrollment, (2) Managed Care product, (3) Health Promotion and Disease Prevention, and (4) Difficult to Cover Services (mental and dental care). Each working group had specific goals that were written into the grant, and over time each group took on its own way of operating.

The Health Promotion and Disease Prevention (HP/DP) working group was led by Sally Findley, clinical professor at the School of Public Health, and Walid Michelen, director of the Ambulatory Care Network, the off-site system of primary care facilities operated by Presbyterian Hospital. This group was truly instrumental in bringing new financial resources and services to the Community Voices partner organizations. The cochairs had a combination of research, public perspective, and hands-on experience with patient care and direct services needs. Sally Findley had a long-standing history with local community organizations in the areas of child health.

The HP/DP working group was sensitive to the fact that the community needed to be brought into the decision-making process on what disease entities should be given priority. Michelen describes the atmosphere this way: "We had no planned project and took nothing for granted. For example, what were the main problems in our neighborhoods? We could spout off a number of the usual diseases, heart disease, asthma, diabetes. But how did we know that this was really the case? Also, we may think that our communities were interested in tackling these issues, but was that really the case? How were we to determine that?"

To answer that question, the group surveyed fifty-nine health care providers and community-based organizations and over seven hundred community residents to determine where to concentrate their energies and then proceeded to move forward on developing and piloting HP/DP initiatives based on the survey. Michelen continues:

> This was a different approach from what most researchers or grantees in either the university or the hospital had done in the past. Usually the principal investigator submits a proposal, with letters of support from the community to a funding agency. After receipt of the funding the P.I. [primary investigator] then begins to recruit subjects/patients for the project. Most projects end once the funding expires. Rarely do CBOs receive any significant funds from the project—and rarely do they hear the results of the research or program. . . . Most CBOs and community residents were skeptical of anything different from that pattern. We wanted to change that perception.

Another working group decided that the mental health issues required a study on which to base recommendations on how to improve mental health care in the community. They involved extensive community-based organizations, the clergy, and community leaders in creating their report (see chapter 12). So, what came about was reflective of the communities' perspectives of the mental health problems they faced. This was a radical departure from past practice in which most academicians decided first what needed to be done and then told the community how to move forward. This change in the framework of collaboration was facilitated by the people who were part of this committee: Charles Corliss from Inwood Community Services, who as cochair of the Northern Manhattan Mental Health Council put the work of the collaborative to the service of this body and in doing so put it "on the map"; Dr. Roberto Lewis-Fernández, a researcher from the New York Psychiatric Institute with a strong background in community engagement; and Drs. Mary McCord and Jennifer Havens, both clinicians with a strong commitment to advocate for children's mental health.

Because each working group addressed a specific health-related area, the members who constituted the working group were involved in that specific area on a day- to-day basis. This allowed the working group to bring service providers, educators, government officials, and researchers to the table based on their areas of interest and expertise. The working group cochairs involved its membership by convening conferences—as was the case with the Mental Health Report—to partner on training of community health workers. One of the goals of the working groups was that all partners benefit from the work of the collaborative. For example, the facilitated enrollment training included frontline staff from the Harlem Perinatal Network, Community Premier Plus, Head Start and Day Care providers, and many others who interacted with local residents to provide services. These individuals were empowered by the training and given the tools to engage residents and learn about new policies and regulations to connect residents with health care services.

By engaging frontline staff at the various organizations, the collaborative played a role in strengthening the organizations' capacity to provide enriched services to their constituencies. Organization staff members were now more aware of how to link people to immunization and disease management programs, such as the Asthma Basics for Children (ABC) initiative, and how to engage in policy and advocacy efforts surrounding health care access issues. Our community partners became valuable assets when we sought to identify the needs as perceived by the community. While many organizations faced limitations in human resources, many felt compelled to engage their staff and get involved in the collaborative's initiatives because they understood the benefits that such involvement yielded. However, as a result of actively getting involved with community-based organizations on a functional basis, the academic and health care partners became aware of the limited resources that the smaller nonprofit organizations had available to engage their staff at various levels of our collaborative. Many of the frontline staff members involved were already working to full capacity and at times extended capacity. Thus, the collaborative continuously explored possibilities for enhanced funding opportunities that would increase our partner organizations' participation across the board.

However, funding initiatives and staff support remained a daunting challenge, with funders requiring new and innovative approaches. The collaborative was saying, "We've found what works: holistic service coordination" among safety net providers and community-based organizations, but funders wanted "new" programs. While the collaborative was successful in tapping into such new programs as ABC, Salud a Su Alcance (SASA), Health Information Tool for Empowerment (HITE), and others (chapters 4, 7, and 8, respectively), there was continual tension between taking on new initiatives and determining more fundamental ways to strengthen the collaborative.

How the Evaluators Viewed the NMCVC

The challenges faced by the collaborative and the working groups became evident in the first evaluation of the NMCVC by outside evaluators. They indicated that there was a need for more coordination between the working groups—a problem of human resources, as many community partners did not have the staff to dedicate to the collaborative's initiatives. The leadership of the NMCVC was aware of the deficiencies of the collaborative early on. In thinking back over the second year of NMCVC, Moisés Pérez said that "we have somewhat dropped the ball, we have not met regularly as we used to and we have not held everyone as accountable as we should have. The collaborative nature of the work is weaker this year than last, but we are still quite vibrant. We need to go back to more regular meetings. And we need to look at all our strategies and evaluate them afresh."

Managing the NMCVC presented a number of challenges for the leadership. A leadership retreat was held to iron out communication issues and project goals and get the team moving in the same direction. Bringing the team, which included the working group chairs and the executive committee, to the university's retreat house, the Arden House in Harriman, New York, provided the opportunity to solidify plans and charge the batteries for the third year of the extensive program.

The outside evaluators, however, noted that "participation in the collaborative activities remains fairly concentrated among the dozen or so who have been involved from the start, but as new programs are launched, more organizations are becoming active members . . . and there are more organizations 'at the table' because it is an important table, not because they receive financial support." In fact, by the final year of the first five years, there were over thirty-five organizations involved in one way or another. Many of them were able to get independent support from having participated in the Community Voices endeavor, and the additional support was, as stated above, quite significant.

This additional support became both a strength and a weakness in keeping the collaboration together. The strength is that the initiative did lead to institutionalizing individual efforts that were undertaken under the Community Voices umbrella. The weakness is that with independent support, the members of the collaborative no longer felt bound to the collaborative and went off in their own directions. By the close of the fifth year, many of the original participants interested in the NMCVC were moving along independently from the collaborative. And as the collaborative moved onto its next phase—four years of funding to undertake advocacy to sustain the efforts in the first phase—only a few of the most dedicated remained consistently involved.

In their final, fifth-year report, the outside evaluators noted the many accomplishments of the NMCVC, along with the key challenges that such collaboratives face:

- Getting people out to meetings
- Funding
- Finding the right staff to work with the community and the university
- Scheduling convenient training times
- Insufficient staff to meet training needs
- Tremendous reliance on volunteers
- Space for conducting programs
- Insufficient time for conducting community work

The report listed several other challenges of keeping members and stakeholders involved in the coalition work, including:

- Competing priorities of churches
- Competing priorities of volunteers, community members
- No reimbursement for time spent in program activities
- No incentives
- No language translation services
- A narrow agenda
- Waning interest as funds dry up

While some of the challenges may seem trivial and others not so, many years of experience have shown that "the devil is in the details." To properly and consistently coordinate activities, the conveners must have the ability to follow up and communicate. It was apparent by the ninth year of the collaborative, with funding running out and many spin-offs from the activities already in place, that interest had waned. However, it was also clear that, as the evaluators pointed out in their final report, the NMCVC had met its goals:

> Since its inception the Northern Manhattan Community Voices has developed a comprehensive collaborative structure linking community-based, faith-based organizations, medical and academic institutions, and safety net providers in northern Manhattan. The initiatives developed by the NMCV have stimulated a more coordinated system of care, improved health coverage, and increased access for the uninsured populations. These efforts have fostered sustainable community-wide health promotion programs for the most threatening and prevalent diseases in northern Manhattan. By bridging existing agencies who served the needs of the community, the NMCV has been able to leverage resources to create effective programs that serve the unmet needs of community residents. The result has been a stronger network of comprehensive health services upon which community residents can rely.

References

New York City Department of Health and Mental Hygiene (2006). *Community health profiles*. http://www.nyc.gov/html/doh/html/data/data.shtml.

Part II

Promoting Health and Primary Care

This part consists of chapters about programs designed to create systems to implement health promotion and disease prevention programs that would enhance community-based primary care. It covers how community health workers became an important part of the workforce that permitted grass roots outreach into the community, and describes a series of specific health promotion programs initiated through the Northern Manhattan Community Voices Collaborative designed to increase asthma control in children, increase the immunization rate in children, and reduce tobacco use.

3

Community Health Workers

A Successful Strategy for Restoring the Health of a Community

MOISÉS PÉREZ, JACQUELINE MARTÍNEZ, and LAURA FRYE

> Community Voices gave us (Alianza) the opportunity to build on what
> we had, a plan for scaling up the work we did, [and] an opportunity to
> reconcile relationships and restore trust among the community and
> the big institutions, like Columbia University.

When I (Moisés Pérez) saw the request for proposals for Community
Voices I thought, "Community Voices, that's us!" It was a perfect match
for Alianza Dominicana, the largest multiservice, community-based organization in Washington Heights. Since I founded Alianza Dominicana in
1987 as a nonprofit community development organization, we had been
working with youth, families, and public and private institutions to
revitalize economically distressed neighborhoods. We were already implementing successful programs that were fueled by our community voices—
voices teaching about pregnancy, voices sharing information about HIV,
voices speaking out against drugs and violence. Our voices were demand-
ing to be heard, and our voices offered tactical, feasible solutions to the
problems facing this community.

So we raised our voices further and became one of the three partners,
along with Columbia University and Harlem Hospital, of the joint application to the W. K. Kellogg Foundation. The grant offered immediate and
dedicated talent that could sit, listen, and plan with us. The support would
allow us to expand the agenda we had been working on and amplify our
efforts to connect our work to a national agenda. And, just as important,
we recognized that the Northern Manhattan Community Voices Collaborative presented an opportunity to reconcile relationships and restore trust

among the community and the big institutions, like Columbia University. Partnering with Community Voices would help reconcile relationships with the very institutions that had seemed to fall silent during our ongoing struggle to reclaim our community.

The mission of Community Voices was to increase access to health care for the underserved. Well, we were certainly underserved and needed access to health care. But we also had a collective vision of health and wellness for the community that stretched far beyond access to a doctor for medical care. It was about the mental well-being of our community residents, the security and safety of our children, and greater educational opportunities for our youth. The NMCVC became an opportunity for us to hone in on multiple topics and plan for comprehensive solutions to the needs of our community.

In this chapter we tell the story of how community health workers (CHWs) became one of the key strategies we used to further our wide-reaching goals. In the initial years, the Health Promotion and Disease Prevention working group, one of the four working groups for the Community Voices Collaborative, focused on three priority health areas: facilitated enrollment for health insurance, child immunization promotion, and asthma management. These three programs became the pilots for the CHW initiative described here. We also describe how Alianza created the Center for Health Promotion and Education to serve as a community hub for insurance outreach and enrollment and numerous health care initiatives. Under the stewardship of Alianza, Community Voices staff formed a working group consisting of other agencies, community leaders, community health workers, university faculty, and health care providers. The CHW initiative, including development of training materials, training workshops, and structure of the program, was developed under the guidance of the working group and integrated into ongoing programs at partner community organizations.

But before we tell that story, we need to tell the story of Washington Heights, the largely Dominican community that lives there, and the birth and early work of Alianza Dominicana.

A Community Under Duress: Internal and External Forces Threaten the Livelihood of Community

During the 1980s and into the mid-1990s, Washington Heights experienced one of its darkest trials, threatening the very fabric of the social, familial, and economic well-being of the community. It started with the decline of jobs during the recession of the 1970s when manufacturing jobs went flying out of New York City in search of cheap labor in other parts of the world. Factories that were once thriving in midtown and employed many of the newly arrived immigrants from the Dominican Republic began to close their doors in the mid-1970s and early 1980s. The ripple effect of a downturn of the economy was also beginning to be felt in ritzy restaurants and hotels that had once flourished in midtown Manhattan and, more important, had been secure places of employment for an upcoming generation of Dominicans that had settled in the northern tip of Manhattan. Little by little, and then faster and faster, families that had come to New York with the promise of that better life began to feel the ill-effects of being a marginalized population that was of value only when jobs that no one else wanted were available.

Yet there remained a remnant of hope in the early 1980s. The early saving graces of this period of economic downturn that would keep the core of the community alive and hopeful were the Dominican-owned bodegas, hair salons, cleaners, restaurants, bakeries, and even day-care centers. The entrepreneurial spirit of the people back in the island had remained a part of them. They worked midnight shifts in the hotels in midtown, in factories or as dishwashers in the elegant restaurants in lower Manhattan, and with their meager savings pooled by entire families and friends, they financed their own businesses back in the Heights. But as the economy continued to worsen, the mid-1980s did not seem so promising.

Washington Heights quickly became the largest, most overcrowded, fastest growing, and youngest community in the state of New York. The school district was the most overcrowded in the state, and there was not a single comprehensive program to support the needs and concerns of a population of young people under the age of 18 estimated at sixty-six thousand. The city simply did not have the resources nor the political will to address the needs of the community. With overcrowded, failing schools, little to no work opportunities, no after-school or recreational programs, a stressed housing stock owned by slumlords, and a host of other ills, the community became a prime candidate for the proliferation of drug sales. While heroin was popular as a drug of choice from the 1950s through the 1970s, the 1980s saw the onset of cocaine use. What started as a fad drug among the wealthy downtown or in New Jersey across the George Washington Bridge seeped in and began to strain the fabric of Washington Heights.

How the creeping dependence on this drug by a wealthy group of white-collar workers and a thriving hobby for a myriad of wealthy kids living across the bridge connected with an army of a younger generation of Dominicans living in the Heights has not been well documented. However, it does not take a sociology degree to connect the dots and figure out how Washington Heights became an epicenter to one of the deadliest drug trades in America. For the younger generation of Dominicans—who were watching their dreams of a better life slowly evaporate, unemployed or turned off by the failing school system—the business prospects were clear. All of a sudden, one year's salary in a factory or one month's income from a bodega could be earned in fewer than five hours—if you were in the right corner at the right time.

But even as the small, yet growing, cadre of local drug dealers was being self-selected into a rising drug business, the majority of residents turned their faces and pretended that nothing was happening. It was easier this way. It was less dangerous. And they were not the only ones in denial. Washington Heights had grown in popularity as an epicenter for drug deals. It was quite obvious to the police department, political leaders, and others in power who could have acted instead of watching passively on the sidelines. The effects of an unchecked illicit industry began to surface pretty quickly and proved devastating to the community. Turf wars became increasingly violent, gunshots became a familiar background noise, and police brutality was becoming more and more visible. All of this ate away at the integrity and resolve of the community and bred more and more fear.

The 1990s brought more trouble. Now it was not the wealthy that were hooked on the white powder—local residents, perhaps ailing from the break-down of their community, began to find solace in the drug. The drug industry found a new market. The task at hand for those in search of profit was to make it more accessible and less expensive. The answer was to transform cocaine into "crack." Now it was a drug less wealthy could afford. This was the drug that would begin to claim hundreds, eventually thousands of lives in Washington Heights. The number of families torn apart because a daughter, son, cousin, nephew, or neighbor was hooked on drugs was steadily growing. Familiar faces were seen in the streets strung out from a high. It had caused an endemic wave of fear of walking in the very streets of a community once known as a home away from home for so many Dominicans.

The fear was crippling. Mothers did not allow their children to walk outside their apartments, and business owners dreaded the evening hours and opted to close earlier, leaving a more fertile ground for isolated streets now dominated by drug businessmen who ruled with terror.

All of these conditions were made worse by years of political neglect by leaders in Albany and in City Hall, and the growing corruption among those charged with the task of keeping the law. The men in blue, New York's Finest, were often associated with the very same people causing havoc in this economically and socially devastated community. A select few police officers had found a niche for themselves and began to benefit financially from the drug industry—setting back any trust built with community residents.

In fact, the community felt completely abandoned and often betrayed by the major institutions. Imprisoned by fear in their own apartments, many would sit before their television sets and hear the evening news tell of the horrific stories of murder, drug raids, and robberies occurring in the community. The question that remained in the minds of people was: Could we ever reclaim our neighborhood? The question was central to any conversation between neighbors, family members, a hair salon owner and their regular customers. Some would say, "Esto no lo arregla nadie" (No one could ever fix this). Underneath the pain, fear, and growing distrust of the authorities, there was a steady heartbeat of hope fueled by a desire to reclaim the streets for the younger generation who had a right to live outside the confines of small apartments.

This was the ailing neighborhood—with an underground and resilient ache for change— in which Alianza Dominicana was born. We, the community members, decided to find that underlying heartbeat and amplify it to drown out all the other noise. We could organize and mobilize with shouts of slogans and feet stomping as we marched forward in search for change—determined to be heard! Washington Heights could surely have used an influx of capital to bolster the dying businesses. It could have benefited from a redoubled effort to reduce crime. Instead it got an even more powerful catalyst of change: a mobilized community. We created an army of our own foot soldiers to attack the problems at hand. This army was composed of leaders from block organizations, churches, tenant associations, and, most of all, those who would later be called "community health workers."

Alianza Dominicana: A New Vision for the Community

Alianza Dominicana (literally translated as "Dominican Alliance") grew out of the determination of the Dominican American community to emerge, flourish, and contribute to the development of American society. The struggles of day-to-day living gave rise to our purpose and challenged us to succeed. We saw a future where Latinos, immigrants, women, youth, and working and poor families were valued contributors to the culture and essential life of our nation. We worked to strengthen communities and affirm the value of family and community life by initiating and implementing programs and services that responded to the full spectrum of community needs and utilized community assets.

The community health workers were the key to this vision. They drove our programs forward, reached out to those people and families who had been marginalized, advocated for necessary change, and shared their knowledge and experience to achieve a wide range of positive health outcomes. We did not label them "community health workers" when we began. (Nor did we know that they were to become central to the success of many of the Community Voices programs—that was all in the future.) At the time, they were part of a team of community members who came from the same class and culture as the people they were trying to reach. They were "ordinary people" who were intricately woven into the fabric of our lives and sought to create a healthier environment, address social issues, improve community leadership, and reclaim hope for future generations.

Years after we began Alianza's CHW initiative, we wrote a paper on the project that was published in the *Journal of Health Care for the Poor and Underserved Community* (Pérez et al. 2006). In the background section of the article, we wrote that

> health workers typically share racial and ethnic backgrounds, cultures, languages, and life experiences with members of the communities in which they live and serve; therefore, they are much better able than people from outside the community to build the trust necessary to succeed and to provide a cost-effective bridge within health care systems and social services. Numerous studies, reports, and experiences in diverse settings show that having CHWs as part of the health delivery system can produce a wide range of benefits, including increased access to care; increased revenue and cost-savings through more effective use of primary

care services; decreased inappropriate utilization, increased appropriate utilization, and improved health outcomes; increased trust between communities and health care providers; and increased flexibility in the health care system.

The Institute of Medicine recognized the importance of CHWs in a 2003 report, stating "Community health workers offer promise as a community-based resource to increase racial and ethnic minorities' access to heath care and to serve as a liaison between healthcare providers and the communities they serve."

Top Priorities: Pregnancy, AIDS, Violence

Teen pregnancy was high, and Alianza's very first funded project as an organization sought to prevent teen pregnancy by mobilizing young people to be leaders within their peer groups and to address sexual health issues. By providing a safe space for young people to unite and using the opportunity to equip them with knowledge and information, we aimed to help young people meet their full potential—before getting pregnant so that when they undertook parenthood, they had all the tools they needed. This task could not have been accomplished by a set of outsiders, coming in and preaching to our youth. It required people with familiar faces and familiar backgrounds, people who could relate to the everyday lives of teens, people who understood the full range of barriers to protecting oneself from precocious pregnancy. A trained cadre of community health workers was the ideal group to undertake this task.

Yet, preventing teen pregnancies was only one part of this larger social concern. We also had women who were experiencing unnecessary risks during their pregnancies because they lacked support as they embarked on parenthood. This led to the creation of Best Beginnings. A group of dedicated community women, trained on early childhood intervention, went into the homes of pregnant women to assess their risk for complicated pregnancies. They would then work with them intensely throughout the pregnancy and birth and stay as a support for the family until the child entered the school system. This home visitation model was completely run by community health workers—women who understood the trials of pregnancy, knowledgeable in the constraints of poverty, and trained to provide the necessary support.

But the layers of the problems confronting this community were thick and many. We had a responsibility, funding or no funding, to collectively identify solutions. As an organization, Alianza could not ignore the epidemic that stole so many of our community members in the late 1980s and early 1990s. AIDS had become another agent claiming the lives of people, and the disease fed on unawareness, fear, and misinformation of the people. We formed a program called AIDSRAP, where our community health workers trained young people in "HIV 101" and theater techniques so they could go forth into the community and talk to other young people about safe sex. They served as the start of a cascade of knowledge sharing through mechanisms that were tailored to the intended audience.

The reproductive and sexual health needs of our community were great, but our conception of health did not stop at these issues. Even more pressing were the drug and violence problems that had imprisoned our communities with fear and relegated us to our homes.

When the doors to Alianza were opened in a New York City Public Housing Authority project on 176th Street and Amsterdam Avenue, there was a crack house right above us on the second and sixth floors. These apartments operated twenty-four hours a day, driving the tenants crazy with the constant incursions. The windows of our future offices had been pulled out to make it easy for addicts to crawl into the warm basement space during the cold winter. The day we moved in to clean up we found a shopping bag of crack vials in the electrical closet (it was the warmest room). We cleaned out our space but could not stop there. We needed to tackle, on a community-wide level, the toughest and most profound dangers facing us: drugs and violence. In our eyes this was the first step in restoring our community, nurturing it back to health, and positioning it for a hope-filled future. It seemed like an impossible undertaking, but the cost of inaction was too great. We were losing too many members of our young and vibrant generation, we were losing hope, and the steady heartbeat for change could easily fade if we did not act fast.

One day I just remember thinking, "Wait a minute, the overwhelming majority of people in this community are horrified at this, but no one is talking!" So I called a community meeting to talk about what we needed to do to address the drug problem. Ten people came. At the time I was so impressed—ten people! At the next meeting we got twenty-five and then fifty, and then, when a critical mass showed up at a weekly meeting, we began to organize a march. On a warm spring day, with a huge group of people, we set out to march from 137th Street up Broadway to 173rd. We pulled together signs, held pictures of our loved ones who had been lost to the drug wars, and carried names of the mothers who had lost a son or daughter to drugs. The media paid attention, and local political leaders such as City Councilmember Stanley Michaels and Maria Luna (the first Dominican to be elected as district leader in New York) heard the cry and demand for change and were willing to join in our efforts to bring about change in Washington Heights.

Another critical moment during this period of mobilization occurred when a young man in our newly formed teen program was killed. His best friend, with whom he grew up and who was engaged to his sister, shot him over a dispute related to drugs. This incomprehensible loss of life spawned Mothers Against Violence—a group that sought to protect the community from this most ultimate public health issue: violence. We sought to draw on the respect and influence of mothers to discuss violence with their children. These mothers also served as community health workers. But the drug problem had to be addressed from several sides. While Mothers Against Violence sought to raise a new generation of children who would peaceably interact, there were drug dealers and addicts on the streets challenging any progress made. We had to create a safe public space for ourselves. We began a project to reclaim Highbridge Park.

We knew Highbridge Park was an environment ripe for drug use, prostitution, and all the behaviors we as a community would no longer accept. We targeted the 180th Street playground and sought help for the seventy-five addicts who lived under the 181st Street underpass. The people of Washington Heights felt empowered to take control—enough was enough. A cadre of women of the community went out, locked the playground, and, taking turns, worked hand in hand to guard it. Parents from buildings close by worked out a schedule to ensure that the entrance was always attended. We did not allow people without children to enter. We called a press conference with some of our elected officials on a hot summer evening, and the following day we were on the phone with the parks commissioner. The Parks Department needed to clean up and restore the park's benches, swings, and play equipment, while we took responsibility for security. Again the city could not ignore the people's voice, and the leaders took notice. The residents of our community were gaining traction. The park was forcibly returned to its original intent—a place for children to play safely and for families to get together and reconnect. It was a small victory to those on the outside but for us it was a major win!

Community Voices: New Opportunities for Organized Change and Development

By the time I (Jacqueline Martínez) joined the leadership team of Community Voices, there was already a common theme woven into these efforts—a commitment for change—built on the strength of community organizations and led by resilient and passionate leadership. Having been born in Washington Heights, with strong familial ties to a large extended family (about thirty-five cousins!), I had witnessed firsthand the audacity of hope and survival among a people who had fought against the ravages of poverty, racism, classism, and marginalization. I saw a willingness to stand up to the fight—both internal and external conflicts—and boldly say no to defeat and yes to hope. There was a powerful force among the people who lived in Washington Heights, and given the right resources, they could collectively reclaim the life of their community. We had individuals who were ready and willing to assume responsibility for Washington Heights and to improve it by doing their part and taking to the street to demand a better neighborhood. The underlying strategy was one of helping those who "wore our shoes" and "walked our path." Mothers who had successful childbirth could teach others about healthy pregnancies, youth doing well in school could tutor their friends, HIV-positive individuals could counsel their peers who were at risk. All of this amounted to a cadre of community residents who understood the power of a collective voice, who would not tolerate the neglect and marginalization of politicians, decision makers, and the large institutions in the community. We had the resources and tools within our community to make it a better place. We would tap into that community heartbeat that been restored and build upon the strengths we already had.

Community Voices evolved on the heels of these victories, presenting Alianza with the means to take the efforts to another level. The "what and how" Community Voices gave the community was the opportunity to figure out a strategy to sustain this movement and bring about change in other areas, plan for scaling up the work we did, and execute a more defined strategy of engage the residents and leaders of our community into health and health care issues.

The Center for Health Promotion and Education

In 1999 an estimated one-third of the population of northern Manhattan was uninsured, yet at least forty-eight thousand residents were eligible for health insurance. Not surprisingly, one of Alianza's early joint efforts with Community Voices was to increase enrollment in public health insurance programs. To that end, we secured a grant from the state to hire and train "facilitated enrollers" for public health insurance programs. (See below for more about this program.) The workforce we had informally trained and dispatched into the streets and homes of Washington Heights became the groundwork for securing this grant. The next step was integrating the idea of enrolling people into health insurance as part of the work we were already doing.

Working with Community Voices as part of the facilitated enrollment program, we began to design the vision for a Center for Health Promotion and Education for the Washington Heights community. With funding from Community Voices and dedicated time to plan, envision, and execute, we designed the blueprint of this center. The next step was securing the location. We took this opportunity to reclaim yet another space that had been taken over by negative forces in our community. A bar/cabaret that hosted degrading wet t-shirt contests operated on the first floor of the building Alianza called home. Having this business in the same building where our youth came for training and tutoring or simply to hang out was distressing to us. After numerous late-night shootings and three homicides in the bar, the police shut it down under a public nuisance law. The landlord was looking for a new bar operator. However, we were determined to step in and eradicate the public hazard. Without any money to pay for the space, we signed a lease. It was in this space that we coordinated a massive, twenty-four-hour humanitarian relief campaign on behalf of the Dominican Republic and Haiti after a devastating hurricane leveled much of these countries. After this campaign, which brought food, medicine, clothing, and supplies to the poor in the Dominican Republic and Haiti, we formally established a home for community health workers and facilitated enrollers. The space had earned the right!

Together with staff and faculty of Community Voices, we wrote training manuals, designed tools for outreach, and created resources for community members to take with them once they walked out our doors. This new center, now decorated with traditional artifacts illustrating the popular

Dominican culture, became a beacon of information, empowerment, and direction for people seeking to live a life to their fullest potential. In keeping with Alianza's "total person approach" and service integration model, our main focus was on training generalists as opposed to experts in one particular health area—whether it was HIV/AIDS, asthma, violence, substance abuse, or diabetes. People's lives could not be separated into pieces; therefore any support we offered could not be done in a fragmented manner.

The center is continuing to work with the university to train community health workers. We joined forces with Sally Findley in her work to support the development of a formalized CHW training program, both through programs and educationally. Findley is now leading the effort to establish a CHW certificate program at the Mailman School of Public Health of Columbia University, right in our backyard. It will be a collaborative program that would ideally allow people to enroll at Columbia or other partner institutions, such as Hunter College, for a curriculum of up to one hundred hours. The program would cover all the core competencies recommended for community health workers, enabling them to compete for jobs.

Facilitating Enrollment in Public Health Insurance Programs

Community Voices was committed to increasing the number of children and families enrolled in public health insurance programs, as a first step to improve the overall health of the community. Community Voices knew that the training of health promoters and enrollment staff was essential to accomplishing this goal. Alianza was able to coordinate a process based on the conviction that the best way to reach underserved communities is to acknowledge their history and culture. Recognizing that a significant number of eligible northern Manhattan residents were deterred from enrolling due to lack of awareness, fears, and experiences of defeat as a result of the bureaucratic labyrinth, Alianza developed a strategy of facilitated enrollment that combined personal attention in a culturally sensitive setting, individual case management, and an integrated approach to the whole family. This strategy enabled Alianza to engage newly arrived Spanish-speaking immigrants in Washington Heights and French- and Creole-speaking immigrants in central Harlem.

We developed our outreach and enrollment training program in 1999. This six-part training series covered not only the steps for screening and facilitated enrollment, but also strategies for effective outreach, communications skills for working with individuals and groups, how to track outreach efforts and to know what is working (and what is not), and role plays on working as a team in a community. The content and the training approach were built on Paolo Freire's theory of critical pedagogy. This Brazilian educator, who based his work on liberation theology, defined education as a function to bring about the "practice of freedom," the means by which men and women deal critically with reality and discover how to participate in the transformation of their world. It was the perfect sequel for the work that organically evolved from Alianza into the work of Community Voices.

Under the Facilitated Enrollment Program we were able to:

- Identify barriers to enrollment
- Revamp existing training materials and standardized enrollment forms
- Centralize the hiring and training of enrollment staff
- Improve the documentation-gathering process
- Create a faster turnaround for obtaining documentation
- Increase the number of applications submitted and approved

As a result, enrollment in Medicaid and Child Health Plus (CHP) increased by 63 percent over the previous year. By 2003 CHWs had facilitated the enrollment of thirty thousand individuals (table 3.1).

Soon after launching its outreach and enrollment project, the NMCVC realized certain individuals and families were more difficult to engage than others. There were many misconceptions about Medicaid and Child Health Plus. These included people assuming that they do not qualify for Medicaid or CHP, that they might be billed later for services they receive, or worse, that Medicaid is a form of "welfare," which they should avoid so as not to be labeled or perceived as dependent on the help of the government. One enroller said: "Many parents still believe that Medicaid is public assistance. They don't want to fill out the absent parent form, or they don't want their children's father to get in trouble. They want to avoid going to the Medicaid office and the lines and dealing with people who don't speak their language. Some actually withdraw because of this. I'd say 8–10%

'disenroll' because of the stigma of being on Medicaid." Another said, "The CHP population is afraid of INS [the Immigration and Naturalization Service]; they want to know the 'catch.' They don't believe it could be free. . . . We have to tell them that there is no need to fear INS and that this is either a free or low-cost plan." Still another said that hardest parts for parents is choosing a doctor and plan for Child Health Plus: "If they just came from Latin America, it is difficult because they don't know any plans or doctors, so they just don't know."

We found that by applying a systematic case management model, even the most difficult individuals and families could be engaged. This model, which was designed to build trust, engages the individual or family first through an outreach worker and then through linking the individual to a facilitated enroller. Because community health workers are often immigrants themselves, they can address the concerns of immigrants about applying for government-subsidized insurance. In addition, rather than just passing out flyers, outreach workers go to schools, after-school programs, adult education centers, immigrant rights programs, health centers, and door-to-door to talk to residents about insurance. Their main job is to engage people and build a level of trust with them. After outreach workers locate individuals in the community who need insurance, they give them an open appointment slip, referring them to Alianza's facilitated enrollment workers. The facilitated enroller then calls the person within twenty-four hours to set up an appointment.

Once the participant decides to apply for insurance, the facilitated enroller screens for eligibility and works with the individual to complete the application. After notification of acceptance, the facilitated enroller continues to work with the participant. This is especially important considering that having an insurance card is not enough to access and use health services. During the first three months, the facilitated enroller calls the family once a month to find out if the beneficiary is using the health system and if not to offer advice and guidance on where and how to begin the process. These follow-up steps are critical, especially since the community health workers are aware of the complexities of a families health and health care needs. For instance, if a child is asthmatic or a family member has a mental health concern, the community health worker can assist the family in identifying the right team of providers for their specific circumstances. After the first three months, the facilitated enroller contacts the participant at six-month intervals. Another main advantage of the follow-up process is that it allows the facilitated enroller to keep track of each individual's date of

TABLE 3.1

Making a Difference: Community Health Workers

PROBLEMS

48,000 uninsured people, including 18,000 children
High asthma, teen pregnancy rates, drugs, and violence
Low immunization rates

SOLUTIONS

Community health workers
A neighborhood health center

RESULTS (AFTER 5 YEARS)

1,504 trained community health workers
30,000 adults and children enrolled in health insurance programs
8,000 immunized children
4,000 families with improved asthma management
A safer playground

recertification. The follow-up calls and visits are also a time when the facilitated enrollers encourage their participants to tell their friends about the Community Voices facilitated enrollment program. This level of contact with the individual builds trust in the community enrollment system, to which the individual turns for continuing advice and administrative assistance.

Throughout all areas of the Community Voices project, but especially in the area of outreach and enrollment, the concept of building relationships of trust with existing service providers was of fundamental importance. Since its inception, we have collaborated with the New York State Department of Health, New York Presbyterian Hospital, and the Greater New York Hospital Foundation, which has enabled us to both sustain and expand our outreach and enrollment efforts.

Inspiration from Far and Near

The national Community Voices program wisely inserted international learning excursions as part of the work to plan and execute programs that would impact an entire neighborhood or city. The opportunity to travel to Latin America to experience the work of community health workers was of transcendental importance in the development of our work. Our staff traveled to Nicaragua, to Trujillo, Peru, and to Colima, Mexico, spending close to two weeks in these communities. The lessons we brought back from these countries helped us widen our vision for the role and function of community health workers as key partners in transforming a community and changing the policies that were working against it.

An anecdote comes to mind. The town of Moche is rich in red soil— so much so that its forebears built the largest mud cities ever conceived on the planet and some of the most beautiful pottery ever produced. During dry and breezy days the air is filled with damaging particles. As a result Moche had a very high incidence of respiratory illness and a number of related mortalities. The local and regional authorities were highly concerned for they had no solutions to the problem. A group of community health workers met to discuss the problem. One noted that when it was really breezy she would pull out her hose and spray her surroundings and that this really helped. Another agreed, noting that she too sprayed, and chimed in suggesting that perhaps this could be done in the entire community. Lacking the resources to do this, they asked for a meeting with the town mayor and made their request. The mayor was intrigued and deployed a water truck to spray the streets of the town during the dry and breezy season as a preventive measure. Within two years the town experienced a dramatic decrease in respiratory illness and no mortalities. Local wisdom won the day. This story confirmed for us that local residents are better able to identify solutions to larger community problems.

The impact of these projects on the health of the public, utilizing very limited material and technological resources and an abundance of humanity, was highly inspiring. The history of community health workers in Latin American countries is deeply rooted in the notion that health is a right and not a privilege. Building and rebuilding broken systems with equity and justice was at the centerpiece of the work of human rights leaders, and educators like Paolo Freire. According to Freire (2003), educational programs can be effective only if they respond to the self-identified priorities of community residents. If people are concerned about illegal drugs and crime, then the window of opportunity for education about health or other issues is around drugs and crime. In addition, Freire advocates education that is applied to solve problems in people's lives. Our exposure to community health workers in these countries deepened our commitment to the implementation of the role of community as key players in policy reform and transformational changes in how health care is to be delivered.

Alianza's integrated outreach and enrollment strategy involves three interacting components: outreach, referral, and facilitated enrollment. The program relies on an integrated team of paid and volunteer workers who are responsible for outreach and facilitated enrollment. The outreach is conducted primarily by community volunteers: high school students, participants in New York City's Welfare Employment Program (WEP), and promotoras. Building on the notion that a satisfied participant will attract more participants, members of the community successfully enrolled in health insurance through facilitated enrollment are asked to help in the effort by becoming community health workers, also known as promotoras, that is to say, residents in the community who promote health insurance enrollment among their neighbors and acquaintances, in their building, among their friends and relatives, and so forth. All the outreach workers speak Spanish, and all live in the northern Manhattan/Washington Heights community. Like the majority of the Washington Heights community, most are either recent immigrants or the children of immigrants, and most are of Dominican heritage. The most effective element of the outreach strategy is the face-to-face outreach contacts made by the promotoras. A remarkable one out of three people contacted through the promotora outreach is successfully enrolled.

By the fifth year of the Community Voices initiative, we had trained a cadre of 1,504 community health workers and established three model programs addressing health and health care needs of the community. The vast majority (98%) of those trained have been women, predominately between 20 and 29 years old. Most have been Latina (67%), and the balance African American. Seventy-three percent live in the community while the rest live in nearby neighborhoods in the Bronx. The community health workers facilitated health insurance enrollment for nearly thirty thousand individuals, assisted eight thousand children to become completely immunized (see chapter 5), and supported four thousand families in improving asthma management (see chapter 4). Although impressive, these figures tell only part of the story. Just as important was the transformative effect the promotoras initiative had on the people in the community and on the community health workers themselves.

During the Community Voices evaluation process, extensive interviews were conducted with many community health workers. They expressed enormous enthusiasm for the work—by the residents because they were so grateful for the insurance to cover their medical expenses, and by the community health workers themselves because, although the work could be quite challenging, they derived much satisfaction from their work. Box 3.1 provides just a few examples.

BOX 3.1

Community Health Workers' Stories

"It's a great relief [to have insurance]. . . . Before, I couldn't make any kind of decisions. Now I can go to any doctor I want, even the best; before, I couldn't. It's like a big weight was taken off of me. In order to cover the hospital costs, I would have had to ask my family in Santo Domingo for money."

"I never had health insurance before because of my status, but now my children have it. Now my child has a regular doctor. At the doctor's office, they treat me like it is regular private insurance."

"There was one older woman that started crying when I asked her if she had insurance. She'd been here about thirteen years and has been very ill. She thought she couldn't get health insurance. I went to her house, brought her here to Alianza, and she got insurance. She blesses me, gives me so many blessings. She says she doesn't know how she can ever pay me for what I have done. This fills me, and makes me feel good."

"Before I came here I felt useless and I would get depressed. Now I feel that I am giving the best of myself. And one gives, not for herself, but for her community. This has been an incredible experience. It has changed my life and my family's life."

"I am supposed to work five hours. Sometimes I am here for more time than that, but I don't even feel it, because it fills me (gives me pleasure) to be here."

"Because of this work I want to study more because one has many opportunities to grow within the work, and to also have a better position."

"I go into the community making housing calls to help people identify and manage asthma, but there are times when you have to do more. . . . A CHW is not just a community member. CHWs are people who want to go to school. To become better. I want to be somebody who can change something . . . to give people the tools to be self-sufficient."

Lessons Learned

Built upon the years of experience working to help rebuild the social fabric and human capital of a community, the most successful elements of this work appear to have been:

- The long history of Alianza in the community and the trust that people have in it as a resource for their families.
- Proactive and culturally relevant training of the staff. People working at the Center for Health Promotion not only are from the community but have received comprehensive training in health insurance and enrollment procedures, cultural sensitivity, and advocacy. The training was meant to empower the workers and the community at large.
- A culturally relevant working environment, in which people feel comfortable and safe, and flexible hours that take into account the needs of working families.
- An integrated outreach and enrollment strategy, with an extensive network of volunteer and paid outreach workers referring insurance inquiries to the trained enrollment staff.
- The satisfied user as a recruiter. This strategy benefits from a burgeoning pyramid of satisfied insured families making referrals to Alianza for insurance and other services.
- Integrating community health worker training and programs into existing community organizations because this approach builds on existing resources and maximizes community assets.
- Going beyond insurance and offering the necessary support and guidance to navigate the health system, use services for timely intervention, and prevent interruptions in care.

Projecting Our Voices Nationwide

Just as the community health workers program transformed the people who were in it, Alianza and Community Voices reached a new stage of maturity and vision. Having accomplished a number of victories in our local neighborhood, the next obvious step for us was to take it to a national platform. Aligning with the goals of the third phase of Community Voices, which we had just secured with an additional grant from the W. K. Kellogg Foundation, I (Jacqueline Martínez) was charged with the task of taking what we had learned and informing a larger audience. One of our most important goals was to sustain the role of community health workers with state and national support. With a strong core of local community health workers, we were in a good position to achieve this goal.

The stages that followed were of research and discovery. While we were collecting our own data and documenting our work, we took on the task of taking the pulse of the rest of New York and other states as it related to community health workers. First, in New York City we began to build relationships with a newly formed group called the Community Health Worker Network of New York City. Together we sought opportunities to collaborate to unite and to organize community health workers from around the city. We cosponsored a citywide conference and funded a survey to take stock of the number of workers in the city, their employers, and funding sources. This market-based analysis was important to us as we aimed to tap into the other financial resources of the state of New York dedicated to improving access and reducing cost.

Energized by our local work in New York City, we then took on the leadership role of documenting the work of community health workers across the country in the eight Community Voices sites. We documented the similarities and differences across sites on issues of training, workforce development, funding sources for CHW programs, and collaborations with community organizations, hospitals, health systems, and universities. Our findings were produced and disseminated to multiple stakeholders.

After this extensive process was completed, we were not quite satisfied that we had found answers to some of our most critical questions: How can we sustain this model of delivering care, addressing social and public health concerns, and increasing access to care? What are the models of reimbursement for the community health workers that most make sense in our fragmented payment system? These questions drove the Community Voices leadership to submit another proposal to the Community Voices National Program Office and the Kellogg Foundation to seek additional support. After successfully securing the resources, we commissioned an assessment of financing mechanisms for community health workers and convened a national conference to bring together thought leaders and decision makers to discuss opportunities to explore funding mechanisms through mainstream sources, like Medicaid and other third-party payers.

We united a core set of leaders to begin formalizing a national community health worker trade association with the goal of organizing the profession at a national level.

Our early stages of research and discovery during the third phase of Community Voices connected us to various movements across the United States aiming to organize, support, and sustain the role of community health workers as part of a larger effort to build a more equitable and accessible health care system. States like California, Texas, Ohio, Minnesota, and Massachusetts, in addition to the Community Voices states (Florida, New Mexico, Colorado, Michigan, Maryland) were leading efforts to strengthen and sustain the role of community health workers. We learned from each of these sites and began to mobilize a national agenda in the United States.

It was time for community health workers from Alianza to spread their wisdom and join forces with other communities throughout New York City and the United States. Washington Heights's community health workers started as the natural answer to the call from a sick community and then developed into a formal model for health promotion complete with a training program. They are the embodiment of what the dedication and spirit of a community can produce.

A New Chapter for Washington Heights

Today, you can safely stroll down 180th street, hearing music playing in bodegas and savoring the tantalizing smell of Dominican cuisine as you turn a corner of St. Nicholas Avenue or Broadway. For the past twenty years, Alianza had led the charge in reclaiming the streets of Washington Heights and unarming the fear that held people captive in their homes, unable to enjoy these simple pleasures.

For ten of those twenty years, we joined forces with the Northern Manhattan Community Voices Collaborative, a local initiative with a national platform and international audience. During those years we built up the infrastructure of the community, organizing the human capital and building a collective vision of a healthy community. Now, another challenge awaits: today, in 2009, we face an economy that has turned downward. The same underlying issues of neglect and marginalization that plunged us into despair in the early 1990s may be at work again.

Yet, we remain hopeful and stand determined that this community, resilient at its core, having survived one of the most violent and destructive periods in its history, will in fact weather the economic recession. The dedication and innovation that birthed the local community health worker programs still exist and are capable of engendering a new solution to today's trials. Challenges remain but, more important, our commitment remains. With a stronger community infrastructure and the same heartbeat pushing us along, we will not slip back to the deafening cries of the 1980s.

References

Freire, P. (1973) *Education for critical consciousness*. New York: Seabury Press.

Howell, E. M., et al. (1998). Back to the future: Community involvement in the Healthy Start Program. *Journal of Health Politics and Policy Law* 23, no. 2: 291–317.

Hughes, D. C., et al. (1997). Integrating children's health services: Evaluation of a national demonstration project. *Journal of Maternal and Child Health* 4: 243–52.

Hunter, J. B., et al. (2004). The impact of a promotora on increasing routine chronic disease prevention among women aged 40 and older at the US-Mexico border. *Health Education and Behavior* 4 (Suppl): 12S–17S.

Levine, D. M., L. R. Bone, and M. N. Hill (2003). The effectiveness of a community/ academic health center partnership in decreasing the level of blood pressure in an urban African-American population. *Ethnic Disparities* 13, no. 3: 354–61.

Lewin, S., et al. (2003). Lay health workers in primary and community health care. *Cochrane Database of Systematic Reviews* 4: 1–103.

Margolis, P. A., et al. (2001). From concept to application: The impact of a community-wide intervention to improve the delivery of preventive services to children. *Pediatrics* 108, no. 3: E42.

Minkler, M., M. Thompson, J. Bell, and K. Rose (2001). Contributions of community involvement to organizational-level empowerment: The federal Healthy Start experience. *Health Education and Behavior* 28, no. 6: 783–807.

Myers, J. (1996). *Kentucky homeplace evaluation*. Hazard: University of Kentucky Center for Rural Health.

National Community Health Advisor Study (1998). *Weaving the future: Final report of the National Community Health Advisor Study*. Baltimore: Annie E. Casey Foundation.

Nemceck, M. A., and R. Sabatier (2003). State of evaluation: Community health workers. *Public Health Nursing* 20, no. 4: 260–70.

Newacheck, P. W., et al. (1995). Decategorizing health services: Interim findings from the Robert Wood Johnson Foundation's child health initiative. *Health Affairs* 14, no. 3: 232–42.

Pérez, M., S. E. Findley, M. Mejía, and J. Martínez (2006). The impact of community health worker training and programs in New York City. *Journal of Health Care for the Poor and Underserved* 17, no. 1 (Suppl.): 26–43.

Ro, M., and H. M. Treadwell (2003). *Northridge Manhattan community health workers and Community Voices: Promoting good health.* Atlanta: Morehouse School of Medicine.

Smedley, B. D., et al. (eds.) (2003). *Unequal treatment: Confronting racial and ethnic disparities in Healthcare.* Washington, D.C.: National Academies Press.

Stuart, M., and M. Weinrich (2001). Home- and community-based long-term care: Lessons from Denmark. *Gerontologist* 41, no. 4: 474–80.

Swider, S. M. (2002). Outcome effectiveness of community health workers: An integrative literature review. *Public Health Nursing* 19, no. 1: 11–20.

Weber, B. E., and B. M. Reilly (1997). Enhancing mammography use in the inner city: A randomized trial of intensive case management. *Archives of Internal Medicine* 157, no. 20: 2345–49.

Witmer, A., et al. (1995). Community health workers: Integral members of the health care work force. *American Journal of Public Health* 85, no. 8 (Pt 1): 1055–58.

Selected Additional References

Alianza Dominicana website: www.alianzaonline.org.

Fullilove M .T., et al. (1998). Injury and anomie: Effects of violence on an inner-city community. *American Journal of Public Health* 88, no. 6: 924–27.

Muldoon A. F. (2004). Washington Heights, New York City. *Global Crime* 6, no. 2: 222.

New York City Department of Health and Mental Hygiene (2006). *Community health profiles.* http://www.nyc.gov/html/doh/html/data/data.shtml.

[4]

Asthma Basics for Children Initiative (ABC)

Building an Asthma Support System from the Ground Up

SALLY E. FINDLEY WITH GLORIA THOMAS, ROSA MADERA-REESE,
MARÍA LIZARDO, MARIO DRUMMONDS, and BENJAMIN ORTIZ

> We must do something about asthma. We can not have another
> asthma death in our community.

One cold day in 1998, a child in a day-care program operated by one of our
Harlem partners died from asthma. While the community was aware of
the problem of asthma, the reaction to this death brought people together
as only a tragedy can. We were already working with the organization to develop an immunization program and the program director said, "We must
do something about asthma. We cannot have another asthma death in our
community." The commitment I (Sally Findley) made to "do something
about asthma" was the beginning of the Northern Manhattan Asthma
Basics for Children Initiative (ABC). This chapter is the story of that
initiative—how it evolved from concern into a multilayered and coordinated program that we hope has made good on that promise of preventing
asthma deaths among the young children of the community.

Defining the Problem

By the mid-1990s the nation's public health practitioners had concluded
that childhood asthma rates were on the rise, and nowhere more sharply
than in the low-income communities of color such as Harlem. In 1997 the
asthma hospitalization rates for children under age 18 were nine per

TABLE 4.1
Making a Difference: Asthma Basics for Children Initiative

PROBLEM: DISPARITIES IN ASTHMA RATES OF PREVALENCE AND HOSPITALIZATION

Percentage of children with asthma symptoms and diagnosis

East Harlem elementary schools: 27%
Harlem day-care centers: 30%
Central Harlem: 30%
United States overall: 6–8%

Asthma hospitalization rates in children under age 18 (per 1,000)

Washington Height/Inwood: 9
Central Harlem: 21
East Harlem: 29
New York City overall: 10

SOLUTION

ABC, a collaborative effort by parents, schools, clinicians, and the community

RESULTS

School absences due to asthma down from 57% to 50%
Emergency department visits down from 71% to 48%
Hospitalization down from 21% to 9%

Sources: New York City Department of Health (2001); Findley et al. (1998); Bonner et al. (2006); Nicholas et al. (2005).

thousand in Washington Heights/Inwood, twenty-one in central Harlem, and twenty-nine in East Harlem; these were well above the equivalent of the overall city average of ten per thousand. But hospitalization rates are only a small share of all asthma, and we needed population-based information, so I joined a team to conduct a survey at two East Harlem elementary schools; we found that 27 percent of the children had asthma symptoms and diagnoses. Others found similar rates in community surveys in Harlem: 30 percent for diagnosed or possible asthma at day-care centers, 29 percent with diagnosed asthma, and 30 percent with possible asthma in the central Harlem zip code of 10026 (table 4.1). These rates were several times higher than the national prevalence rates of 6–8 percent. In 1998 I led the effort by the Health Promotion and Disease Prevention working group to identify health problem priority areas, and these surveys and conversations found that asthma was consistently among the top five health problems identified by over seven hundred residents of northern Manhattan. For many, addressing asthma was their top priority.

The national medical community responded to the asthma epidemic by reviewing and updating the guidelines for asthma diagnosis and management. The problem was *not* that we did not know how to manage asthma, but rather that we did not do a good a job of ensuring that children actually received all the elements of recommended care, both medical and home asthma management activities. In New York City—as well as the rest of the United States—physicians were not applying the guidelines to their diagnosis and medical management practices, underprescribing corticosteroids and providing little written guidance to patients for home management of medications. Parents received far too little coaching on how to properly adjust medications in case of an exacerbation. They also were not instructed about removing items in the home that trigger their child's asthma. More was needed than simply giving physicians information on state-of-the-art asthma management. Innovative strategies were needed to educate and guide patients so that they could successfully reduce their risk of serious asthma exacerbations. We also wanted to make sure that we reached all children, including those with asthma symptoms who were not yet diagnosed and those who did not have a regular primary care physician. All signs pointed to the need for a collaborative effort by parents, schools, clinicians, and the community.

Thus, when we began exploring the type of asthma program that would work best in our community, we concluded that the most promising programs to improve asthma management were community-based, involving a partnership of medical providers, parents, and the institutions able to work with parents through a variety of channels.

Listening to the Community

We began by talking with 145 community leaders, teachers, and parents. In box 4.1, their words reflect the main themes touched upon in these discussions.

BOX 4.1
In Their Own Words: Community Leaders, Teachers, and Parents

Respond to the parents' desire for a better future

"There's a deep longing for better among parents, for more—for the next generation of parents and primary care givers. I cannot think of a parent or guardian who does not say 'I want more for my children, than I have for myself.'"

"Bring more information to the parents. Inform the people about their rights about the environment . . . and how to advocate for better places."

Work with parents through community organizations

"There are some mothers that don't know about asthma and need help."

"Only as parents become empowered, can children benefit."

"We need to get people involved, in whatever language, so they feel part of it, we need to start from there. . . . That's the important role of community organization; there's a great excitement in becoming part of wider society, of the greater spark. The community is cells coming together and working together, overlapping circles of strength."

Train leaders within the community

"You need leadership. . . . We need to have qualified people, and we need to give support to the people of the community. Part of the credit of this community is the commitment by people who want to give back, and that is still a strength today."

"You need lots of information, lots of resources. You have to be able to tell them what the options are, regarding neighborhood resources for any situation that might come up."

Provide options and choices

"We have always had a commitment to people, to provide a wide spectrum of choice."

"It is not that we don't care. We do. We are so busy. Please make it easy for us to participate in the program. Not too long or during the day when we work."

(Continued)

BOX 4.1 (*Continued*)

Incorporate asthma education into community programs

"The message about trigger reduction is often missed in doctor's visits, and community groups can get this message out. Checklists help organize the search for triggers."

Help parents get more out of the doctor's visits

"It was hardest when I was running to the emergency room without knowing what was going on. The doctors should tell us sooner about asthma."

"The doctors send the medical forms with the children when they come to the daycare and they say the children are okay. . . . Sometimes I see symptoms but the doctor didn't say that the child has asthma. So I tell them [the parents] to work with the doctor and ask questions."

"I did not know how to ask the doctor. I was not aware of the controller medication and side effects. . . . I did not know that you need to give children the medication regularly."

Help people organize the information

"The handbook concept, having everything in one place, meshes well with our desire as teachers to educate and share knowledge. It empowers us to speak about asthma one-on-one with parents, because the handbook supports our message."

"There is a take-home message that goes with the handbook. Questions about asthma management don't arise just at a training; a handbook can be there to help when the question comes up well after the training."

Guiding Principles into Action

At the end of the exploratory period, we had a name and a mission: Northern Manhattan Asthma Basics for Children (ABC), with the mission of reducing the burden of living with asthma for all children under age 12 in the community through a partnership of community organizations, schools, and health care provider networks. I was asked to take on leadership of the coalition, given my leadership in the exploratory period and my previous work to address the problem of asthma in the community. We adopted the following guiding principles:

- Parents come first, putting parents in charge
- By the community, for the community
- Integrating asthma education into community programs
- Community health workers work with parents
- Diverse options for working with parents, but all using materials selected and/or developed by the coalition
- Reaching out to the providers to improve communications
- Make it fun for children, teachers, and parents

Parents Come First

We heard from parents and organizational leaders loud and clear about their concern to be able to take care of their children with asthma, so we adopted the principle of "Parents come first" for ABC. We convened a parent advisory board with parents from each of the partner organizations and participating day-care centers. The parent advisory board translated the ABC mission into the following aim: to transform parents' love and concern into effective asthma care for their children. "Parents come first" is consistent with the movement in the medical community toward patient-centered care. We incorporated parent and child education components from the national inner city asthma program. We also incorporated the principles of popular education articulated by Paolo Freire, namely, that people learn when they care about the problem and are engaged in addressing it.

By the Community, for the Community

The coalition's next guiding principle is "By the community, for the community," meaning that we used community-based decision processes, recommended as key to achieving effective and sustainable programs. Programmatic decisions, small and large, were made by the coalition, using consensus processes and guided by our parent advisory board. This maintained a balance in the academic–community partnership making up the coalition. The community medical providers served as advisors and partners in improving asthma care, not the lead decision makers. While Mailman School of Public Health housed the coalition, we at Mailman did not run it.

The principle of "By the community, for the community" was translated into a decentralized management structure. While we at Mailman School of Public Health had overall responsibility for evaluation, reporting, and, importantly, fund-raising, two community organizations led the coalition's activities at the two main activity hubs, Northern Manhattan Improvement Corporation for Washington Heights/Inwood and Northern Manhattan Perinatal Partnership for Harlem. These hubs split the management and oversight for all the participating programs: thirteen community programs, thirty-one day-care centers, ten schools, and two community pediatric practice networks. Each organization discussed with their hub leader their targets for ABC activities and obtained support for those activities through a subcontract with the hub organization. Enrollment and participation targets varied with the size of the program, but typically ranged from 40 to 140 families of children with asthma per site.

Integrating Asthma Education into Community Programs

We opted for integration of the asthma educational programs into ongoing educational and community development programs, rather than a stand-alone program or one based out of the hospital or clinical system. This principle of integration also was consistent with our vision of building on the community assets and strengths. One of the founding members of Community Voices and leader of the Adair Community Life Center, Thelma Adair, said, "Community is both now and future—and that's the strength of working with community: it's a foundation stone to build on. New initiatives can flourish quickly when they can anchor themselves in unsung, unknown heroes; these are the informal structures that can be tapped into, the human resources."

Because we were interested in children under age 12, we decided to work with the programs that educate our youth. How were programs to integrate asthma-related activities into their activities? Each partner program agreed to incorporate the following activities into their programs:

1. Identify children with asthma using asthma questions on enrollment or medical forms.

2. Engage parents of children with asthma in asthma educational activities.
3. Facilitate parent–primary care provider communication about asthma.
4. Engage *all* children in asthma educational activities.
5. Make the organization asthma-friendly.

We designed our training and support to enable teachers and staff at each organization to offer these program elements in their routine work with parents and children. We included basic asthma signs and symptoms screening questions with the medical forms required for registration for school or day-care programs, and we adapted this screening process for all the programs. We developed activities and games for teachers to add to their health units. We developed a parent educational program that could be offered by core coalition staff or by the teachers or social workers at each program. Working with our partners, we developed processes for doing environmental assessments and worksheets for guiding staff or parents in reducing triggers. We then developed a set of training materials, the ABC Handbook series, to guide center or school staff in implementing the program, as well as a complementary handbook for parents.

We established an organizational partnership process to make it as easy as possible for the organization to fulfill its dream of an asthma program for the parents. A critical first step was to identify the key individual(s) charged with liaison with ABC and carrying out asthma-related activities at the program. We provided different program options for engaging staff, parents, and children in asthma educational activities, and we established a calendar for accomplishing the activities.

Community Health Workers Work with Parents

Our program leadership was firmly committed to community health workers for the critical work of engaging parents in asthma self-management education. In our exploratory interviews community and organizational leaders had advocated for training their own staff to become leaders, and this preference was strongly supported by evidence of the effectiveness of community health workers. We therefore built our program around community health workers, adopting a broad definition for community health worker, including both educators and case managers who add asthma activities to their routine teaching or social work responsibilities as well as those who integrate asthma activities into activities solely focused on health issues. We developed a training program to give community health workers the skills needed. The *ABC Early Childhood Educator Handbook* and the *ABC Parent Handbook* were developed as core tools guiding community health workers in their work with parents. Both handbooks and all our educational videos and materials were produced in English and Spanish, so that community health workers and parents could work in either language.

Community health workers were recruited from among the staff (teachers, social workers, family visitors, case managers) and parents of children with asthma. We had a variety of niches available in the program, and we adapted the training to the roles and responsibilities of the particular niche. The basic training was completed in four hours, but additional training of up to forty-eight hours was provided to enable community health workers to perform additional roles. The evaluations conducted before and after the training showed there was an 83 percent increase in knowledge of asthma. In our annual feedback surveys, those trained said that they learned a great deal from the training. Importantly, the child-care providers reported that they now knew how to handle asthma and how to work with parents. In box 4.2, teachers and day-care providers tell us how they applied what they learned at the workshops.

Parent Empowerment

Our approach has been to start where the parent is at, giving space for expression of fears and doubts. We helped parents see how taking care of their children's asthma is an extension of their basic role of protecting and nurturing their children. We worked with parents to help them express and then address their fears of the daily preventive or controller medications. We next showed parents how to be prepared for managing their children's asthma. Through workshops, one-on-one discussions, video presentations, and group discussions, we discussed asthma basics, medications, asthma action plans, triggers, and going to the doctor. We showed parents where to look in the *ABC Parent Handbook* for answers to their questions. For example, we showed them where to find a list of questions that their doctor might ask, as well

BOX 4.2

In Their Own Words: Teachers and Day-Care Providers

"I didn't know anything. I learned a lot. I learned to avoid the triggers, to have the children get tested to see if they are allergic to certain triggers and what affects them, and to see which symptoms they have. . . . I learned how to work with the child who has asthma and recommend to parents that they go to the doctor and get medications."

"Before I didn't have enough information to know how to care for children with asthma. Now, I can help our parents to understand better and how to deal with asthma if they have a child with it."

"I ask the mothers questions about the children. I ask how bad is the asthma, how does she see the condition of the child, because each child is different. I get her daytime phone numbers and an emergency number— and have a plan with her. I ask if she has to give the child medications, which ones, and for the letter from her to give permission to care for the child if the child becomes sick."

"They gave me a video from *Sesame Street*—I put on the videos. They are very good. They tell about what the environment has to do with asthma. They tell the children that you can't have pets. They tell them that they can have fish, because those don't trigger asthma. The handbook is a guide that can be used. I keep the handbook on my desk. It is my asthma 'bible.'"

as questions that they might want to ask, such as "How bad is my child's asthma?" or "Why does my child need to take medicine even when she is feeling fine?" Finally, we ended with a long discussion about environmental triggers of asthma and gave them a Trigger Checklist to use to identify what might be affecting their child's asthma. We gave them room-specific Trigger Worksheets to guide cleanup activities in the bedroom, living room, kitchen, and bathroom. These workshops were offered in one two-hour or two one-hour segments, depending on scheduling preferences of the organizations.

Asthma care has changed since we first developed the handbook, and with the release of the 2007 revision to the national asthma care guidelines, we updated the handbooks. This was an extensive revision, incorporating suggestions from the many staff and parents using the handbooks, the parent advisory board, and community physicians. We also reorganized and simplified the material, both shortening it and making it more accessible to low-literacy users. Finally, in keeping with our electronic age, we are now making the revised handbooks available on the Internet, through the Harlem Health Promotion Center website, www.gethealthyharlem.org.

We tracked how parents applied what they learned with an annual feedback survey to a sample of parents who have participated in the program and with a follow-up survey conducted at the end of the school year (1,108 completed as of this writing). These tracking procedures were part of the protocol approved by the Columbia University Medical Center Institutional Review Board.

Like the staff, the parents gave uniformly positive feedback on the program. They reported using the program's information when they went to the doctor, as well as in addressing triggers in their homes. Box 4.3 provides a sampling of what the parents said in the feedback surveys.

Diverse Options for Parents

The parents and organizations requested flexibility and options, and we therefore developed a variety of tools and options for member organizations. In addition to the *ABC Parent Handbook*, we added a "welcome package" with basic information about asthma and an invitation to participate in ABC, given out at the beginning of the school year to all parents whose child had asthma symptoms or diagnosis. We organized workshops at times convenient for the organization and parents, often in the evenings, but also about the time they were dropping off their children for school. Periodically, the parent asthma mentors set up a table in the center or school hallway where they could be available to respond to questions about asthma or ABC. We tried to integrate our educational sessions into parent–teacher events, and we frequently set up the video to do a continuous showing of *Roxy to the Rescue* at a time when parents came to the center or school.[1] We were on hand at these showings to respond to questions parents had about their own children's asthma. In addition, we held regular asthma educational sessions at community locations and at some of the largest community pediatric practices.

At the request of the parents and staff that we do more for the children with the most severe asthma problems, we developed a care coordination

BOX 4.3
In Their Own Words: Parents

Knowing about asthma

"My son had problems breathing all the time in Mexico, and the doctor said it was flu. But when he got sick here, the doctor said it was asthma. She explained it to me, but I didn't understand. When I heard about the ABC program, I came to a workshop. They explained everything. Now my son takes the medicine and isn't sick all the time anymore."

"When my child first had an asthma attack, it was scary and I did not know what to do. But now I am able to know when the attacks are coming. Oh what a difference!"

Gaining confidence in managing asthma

"I now give Singulair to my four year old, and since I started using it he hasn't gotten asthma. At the beginning I felt bad because I didn't know what to do, and now I feel good because I do."

"It's good to know what to do. My son was 7 months old when he got asthma. It was very difficult and it was a very bad experience for me. I wasn't sure if he was going to live. He's now 4 years old and I am a mother who now knows what to do. . . . I feel sure of what I do and how I treat him."

"I learned to have confidence in myself when my daughter has asthma. I try to be calm and react better so I can manage my child's asthma and help her. The training helped me to spot her asthma signs and know what to do."

"This information helps us to not be afraid and to know what to do in the future. It taught us to take steps needed to prevent on time."

Asking the doctor questions

"They teach us how to ask the doctor. I think that is important because we do not know what are the consequences of the medications in children, now we can ask the doctor about it."

"I've used the information to ask doctors questions."

"They explained asthma to me with more detail than the doctor tells me."

"The training helped me to follow the treatment plan the doctor gave me, because before I was doing the treatment the wrong way."

program to offer one-on-one consultation, education, and assistance. The care coordinators made home visits to assist families in assessing their home environment and offered assistance in getting them started on reducing triggers. We teamed up with a group of community pediatric providers at the Morgan Stanley Children's Hospital of New York and Harlem Hospital to offer this service to high-risk children who have had frequent, serious asthma exacerbations requiring hospitalization or repeat visits to the emergency department. Families received phone calls and home visits at least monthly for the first six months, and then follow-up calls for another six months. During these visits, the family asthma workers covered the same topics as in the ABC workshops, but the discussions were tailored to the individual family needs. Each family received at least one home visit, and these were critical turning points for the families in gaining control of their home environment. More than five hundred families have benefited from these services, and many have become proud graduates, confident in their ability to manage their child's asthma.

Reaching Out to Medical Providers

To help parents get more out of their visits to the doctor, we also developed a set of programs for community pediatric providers, offering training and support aimed at improving the way they managed asthma in their practices. We adopted the Physician Asthma Care Education program (PACE) because it was effective in the areas of greatest concern to us, namely, improvement of communications between parents and physician, with positive outcomes for children's asthma management. PACE is a four-hour training program, using materials developed by the PACE team at the University of Michigan. Seven ABC collaborators (two pediatric pulmonologists, three pediatricians, and two behavioral scientists) were trained to offer the program. Beginning in 2005 we jointly sponsored this training with the New York City Department of Health and Mental Hygiene (DOHMH) to offer four CME units to attendees.

Based on feedback received from the first set of session evaluations, we adapted the training program to include a more culturally appropriate role-play of a physician preparing an asthma action plan for a mother with an active 4-year-old at her side; more information about asthma practice or teaching aids available either from ABC or the DOHMH, invitations to send referrals of patients for care coordination to high-risk children, offers to conduct patient education sessions in their offices, and, of course, distribution of the *ABC Parent Handbook* for use with their patients. In the past year, for example, ABC distributed over four hundred handbooks (English and Spanish) to community providers. We followed up with the providers two to four months after their training to ascertain how their asthma management practice had changed.

Make It Fun!

Our last guiding principle was "Make it fun!" We wanted to destigmatize asthma for both parents and children. To that end, we included games, activities, and videos for all children, regardless of their asthma status. These covered basic asthma concepts: (1) signs of asthma; (2) what to do if you or your friend has trouble breathing; (3) asthma triggers and how to remove them; and (4) asthma medications and when to use them. As noted above, day-care teachers were provided with activity units suggesting games and other materials that they could include in their health units. For the past five years, ABC has sponsored a World Asthma Day poster competition. The posters are professionally judged, and awards are given out at a festive ceremony, generally held the last week of school. The ceremony has evolved into a community celebration with up to three hundred people in attendance, with parents proudly photographing their children as they receive the awards, and everyone generally celebrating what they have accomplished during the year. The award-winning posters are displayed in the subsequent school year at participating schools and selected New York City art galleries. Beginning in 2007, ABC and its partner WIN for Asthma (based at Children's Hospital of New York) have sponsored an asthma walk in the Washington Heights/Inwood neighborhood. This past year more than 150 children and families attended the ABC/WIN for Asthma Walk, ending with a joint celebration with the Climb the Heights birthday celebration at Dyckman Avenue.

ABC in Action: Putting It All Together

Every year the coalition assesses how well we are doing in reaching our goals of improved asthma management for children under age 12 in northern

Manhattan. We look at reach, participation, behavior change, and asthma outcomes.

Reach

By June 2008 we were working with fifty-five different community programs: thirty-two Head Start and day-care programs, ten schools (pre-K–fifth grade), five parenting programs at multiservice community organizations, three faith-based community children's programs, two housing advocacy and tenancy groups, and three family assistance programs, such as the Special Supplemental Nutrition Program for Women, Infants and Children. All participating sites had staff trained, including virtually all teachers and aides at the day-care centers and half the teachers at the elementary schools. Half the centers and schools had designated a parent asthma mentor by school year 2008. By June 2008 ABC had trained 1,412 staff and volunteers. Over half (55%) of those trained were day-care teachers and 31 percent were school teachers, who were perhaps for the first time taking on the role of community health workers. In addition, 14 percent were parents trained into one of the alternative community health worker niches. Most centers or schools (76%) had conducted an assessment of asthma triggers on their premises, and most of them (71%) had taken steps to reduce triggers. Well over half (58%) had sponsored at least one ABC workshop for parents.

Community Provider Participation

Also by June 2008, we had trained 276 out of 306 pediatric primary care providers in our community. The training led to changes in their asthma management practices. They were more likely to use the recommended asthma management tools and skills. The greatest increases were in regular classification of asthma severity, from only 35 percent prior to the training to 83 percent after the training. Appropriate use of controller medications for children with persistent asthma increased from 61 percent to 95 percent. Physicians also reported an increase in their introduction of the topic of environmental triggers, from 5 percent prior to the training to 41 percent after completion.

Participation by Parents and Children

We are now working at capacity, reaching approximately 2,600 children per year in the day-care program, over half the licensed group day-care slots in northern Manhattan, and we reach about 4,000 children per year through our partnership with elementary schools. Half of the children at school have participated in the asthma screening. Across all five years, a total of 33,289 children were eligible for screening, and 16,590 parents returned the screening forms (50%). Of those who returned the forms, 18 percent of their children had symptoms and diagnosed asthma and 17 percent had possible asthma, based on symptoms. Given that completion of the ABC screener is voluntary, the 50 percent response rate sustained throughout all our sites speaks for the interest of parents in the program. The rates are higher in the day-care setting (over 70%), where the individualized intake process increases the response rate.

Between 2003 and June 2008, 4,010 or 70 percent of parents eligible to participate in the program participated in at least one ABC activity, and 2,644 or 66 percent of these participating parents took part in two or more activities. When we recognize how busy the parents are in the community, these participation rates suggest that our strategy of integrating the asthma-related activities into ongoing programs in which the parents were already participating made a difference. We also heard from the parents that they liked the different options—particularly the video, which was short, entertaining, and very informative.

With their training in leading asthma games and activities, the teachers introduced 1,913 children to asthma basics. Between 2004 and 2008, 3,335 children submitted posters for the ABC World Asthma Day poster competition, and more than two hundred families participated in the asthma walk led by ABC and WIN for Asthma in 2007 and 2008.

Behavior Change by Parents and Children

Parents who participated in the ABC program demonstrated significant changes in their asthma awareness and confidence in managing asthma. These changes are reflected in their feedback to the program, which is replete with their newly gained confidence in going to the doctor, seeing the signs of an impending asthma attack in their child, using medications appropriately, and managing the attacks when they do come. The impact of the program is also evident in the changes in asthma management behavior reflected among the parents who reported using the *ABC Parent Handbook*. We have end-of-school-year follow-ups from 1,133 of the parents participating in the program, and among these 25 percent reported specifically that they had used the handbook. We compared the changes in asthma management behaviors for those who used the handbook against those who did not report on using it. As shown in figure 4.1, those who used the ABC handbook were significantly more likely to demonstrate the recommended asthma management practices. Most (93%) of those who reported using the handbook found it easier to talk to the doctor about their child's asthma, and 90 percent said that they were usually or always confident that they could manage their child's asthma. Almost all (96%) of those using the handbook knew their child's asthma triggers, and 91 percent had done something to reduce their child's exposure to these triggers. Over half (60%) had obtained an asthma action plan from their child's doctor, and 47 percent had brought the plan to the child's school. The high proportion of parents obtaining asthma action plans from their child's physicians is evidence of their proactive interactions with physicians. Equally remarkable is the fact that almost half of all parents actually brought the plan to the center or school. This reflects the combined pressure from the parent and the center. The workshops and handbook encourage the parent to bring a copy of the plan to their child's school and

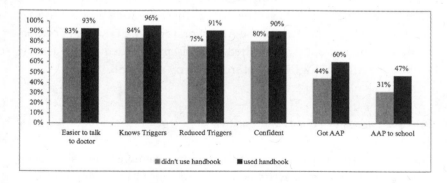

Figure 4.1   Change in Parents' Asthma Management Practices by Use of ABC Handbook

Note: Chi-square tests for these comparisons all have p values <.01

explain why this is beneficial for them and their child. In addition, the program encouraged all centers and schools to be more proactive in requesting asthma action plans from all children with asthma.

The gains in the partner organizations' asthma awareness, improvements in community physicians' asthma practices, and positive shifts in the parents' asthma management behaviors are all reflected in changes in children's asthma experiences. Before participating in the program, the children demonstrate a high level of asthma morbidity, particularly among those who already have an asthma diagnosis. Among the 1,441 with diagnosed asthma, 58 percent had missed school days in the previous month due to asthma. In the past year, 71 percent of those with diagnosed asthma had been to the emergency department for their asthma, and 21 percent had been hospitalized. Half (50%) were on controller medications. After participating in the program, the children with diagnosed asthma had significant reductions in the burden of their asthma. As shown in figure 4.2,

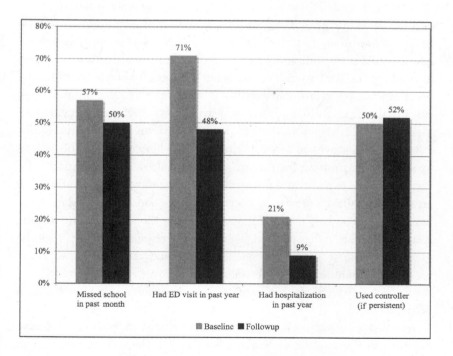

Figure 4.2   Children's Asthma Status Before and After Participation in ABC (Diagnosed children only)

after participating in the program throughout the school year, the 551 children with diagnosed asthma whose parents completed ABC follow-up interviews were less likely to report absences due to asthma in the previous month, significantly down from 57 percent to 50 percent. In addition, those who participated in the program had huge and statistically significant reductions in visits to the emergency department, down from 71 percent to 48 percent, and hospitalizations for asthma, down from 21 percent to 9 percent. The only asthma management indicator that changed little after participation in the program was appropriate use of controller medications among those with persistent asthma, which was 50 percent at baseline and 52 percent at follow-up, not significantly different.

The Road Ahead

We are very proud of these accomplishments. We know we still have a ways to go to meet our goal of enabling *all* parents in the community to have confidence in managing their children's asthma, but if the feedback we have received is any indication, continuation of our current activities is likely to get us there. We have not yet analyzed the impact of our care coordination program, but preliminary feedback from parents in this program suggests that care coordination will help drive down the emergency department visits and hospitalizations to our goals. We are also continuing our follow-up with providers in the community and anticipate that this follow-up will further improve their management practices, and particularly how they prescribe, explain, and follow children on controller medications, an area where we have not been as successful as we had hoped. Updating the handbook and putting it on the Internet will give the providers and parents a common tool that they can use together in the physician's office. With the guidance of our trained staff, teachers, and community health workers, we will facilitate access to the website at day-care centers, schools, and community libraries, so that parents have the information they need on demand.

Our program was born out of concerns by day-care providers, and we believe that the program is working very well in these sites. Steps taken by the New York City DOHMH to include asthma screening questions in the medical forms required for enrollment in child-care programs now means that we no longer need to do screening, but we do need to make sure that day-care providers use this information to reach out to parents with symptomatic or asthmatic children. Trainings offered by the Asthma Training Institute of the DOHMH could be offered to day-care providers, much as the department currently offers training on promotion of physical activity.

We also need to make further improvements to our program with schoolchildren. The various and bureaucratic complexities associated with different departmental authorities (Department of Education and DOHMH), regional school districts, and individual school differences have impeded communication about asthma among the many relevant persons at the schools. Working with the Healthy Schools, Healthy Families network in seven of our ten schools has helped to cut through some of these problems, as has appointment of a parent asthma mentor to work directly with parents. But we can do more. We need to develop an improved way of communicating about children with asthma, so that the nurses, principals, and ABC all are working from the same lists and able to share information without continual fear of privacy violations. We need to be more creative about using available school-based programs, such as Open Airways. We have begun organizing Open Airways trainings for students with asthma at participating schools, but to date we are only able to include the children whose parents have completed the school's medication administration form, which is only a small fraction of all children with asthma at the school. We need to find ways to make the program addressing asthma education more inclusive of all children at the schools, just as we have at day-care centers. This is what we do with the poster competition, and it is the model for how we want to proceed with Open Airways trainings. Reaching more parents, especially of children in elementary schools, should be facilitated by our expanded ABC website, but we will still need to work with parents to spread the word about the website and demonstrate its use. Finally, we hope that we will be able to incorporate more interactive features that will be helpful for both the children and their parents. With the structural changes already laid down for identifying children with asthma and engaging them in asthma educational activities through day-care centers and schools, we believe that these additional changes will bring us within reach of our goal of helping all parents transform their love for their children into the very best asthma care possible, a partnership of the child, parent, schools, and physicians.

Note

1. This 3-D animated video helps adolescents and children cope with asthma and comply with treatment. It covers the nature of asthma, warning signs, triggers, and self-management.

References

Bonner, S., et al. (2006). Oral B-2 agonist use by preschool children with asthma in East and Central Harlem, New York. *Journal of Asthma* 43: 31–35.

Butz, A. M. (1994). Use of community health workers with inner-city children who have asthma. *Clinical Pediatrics* 33, no. 3: 135–41.

Cabana, M. D., B. E. Ebel, et al. (2000). Barriers pediatricians face when using asthma guidelines. *Archives of Pediatrics and Adolescent Medicine* 154: 685–93.

Cabana, M. D., K. K. Slish, et al. (2006). Impact of physician asthma care education on patient outcomes. *Pediatrics* 117, no. 6: 2149–57.

Centers for Disease Control and Prevention. (2002). Surveillance for asthma, United States, 1960–1999. *Morbidity and Mortality Weekly Report* 51(SS-1): 1–13.

Clark, N. (1989). Asthma self-management education: Research and implications for clinical practice. *CHEST* 95, no. 5: 1110–13.

Clark, N. M., M. Gong, M. A. Schork, D. Evans, et al. (1998). Impact of education for physicians on patient outcomes. *Pediatrics* 101, no. 5: 831–36.

Clark, N. M., M. Gong, M. A., Schork, L. A. Maiman, et al. (1997). A scale for assessing health care providers' teaching and communication behavior regarding asthma. *Health Education and Behavior* 24, no. 2: 245–56.

Clark, N. M., and N. J. Schneidkraut Starr (1994). Management of asthma by patients and families. *American Journal of Respiratory and Critical Care Medicine* 149: S54–S56.

Evans, D., et al. (1997). Improving care for minority children with asthma: Professional education in public health clinics. *Pediatrics* 99, no. 2: 157–64.

Findley, S. E., K. Lawler, et al. (1998). "Prevalence of Asthma among Different Ethnic Groups of School Children in a High-Risk Urban Neighborhood." Paper presented at the American Public Health Association Meeting, Washington, D.C.

Findley, S. E., et al. (2003). *The Asthma Solutions Handbook for Early Childhood Educators*. New York: Trustees of Columbia University and Asthma and Allergy Foundation of America.

—— et al. (2003). *Helping Your Child Live with Asthma: A Parent's Handbook*. New York: Trustees of Columbia University.

Fisher, E. B., L. K. Sussman, et al. (1994). Targeting high risk groups: Neighborhood organization for pediatric asthma management in the Neighborhood Asthma Coalition. *CHEST* 106, no. 4 (Suppl.): 248S–59S.

Fisher, E. B., R. C. Strunk, L. K. Sussman, C. Arfken, et al. (1996). Acceptability and feasibility of a community approach to asthma management: The Neighborhood Asthma Coalition (NAC). *Journal of Asthma* 33, no. 6: 367–83.

Fisher, E. B., R. C. Strunk, L. K. Sussman, R. K. Sykes, and M. S. Walker (2004). Community organization to reduce the need for acute care for asthma among African American children in low-income neighborhoods: The Neighborhood Asthma Coalition. *Pediatrics* 114, no. 1: 116–23.

Freire, P. (1973). *Education for critical consciousness*. New York: Seabury Press.

Friedman, A. R., et al. (2006). Allies' community health workers: Bridging the gap. *Health Promotion Practice* 7, no. 2 (Suppl.): 96S–107S.

Lewis, M. A., et al. (1996). Organizing the community to target poor Latino children with asthma. *Journal of Asthma* 33, no. 5: 289–97.

Luis, E. Z., R. Carlos, R., Jaen, and K. Michael (1999). Exploring lay definitions of asthma and interpersonal barriers to care in a predominantly Puerto Rican, inner-city community. *Journal of Asthma* 36, no. 6: 527–37.

Margolis, P. A., et al. (2001). From concept to application: The impact of a community-wide intervention to improve the delivery of preventive services to children. *Pediatrics* 108, no. 3: 42.

Meurer, J. R., et al. (1999). The Awesome Asthma School Days Program: Educating children, inspiring a community. *Journal of School Health* 69, no. 2: 63–68.

National Institutes of Health. (1997). *Guidelines for the diagnosis and management of asthma*. No. 97–4051 Expert Panel Report 2. Bethesda, Md.: National Asthma Education and Prevention Program, National Heart, Lung and Blood Institute.

National Institutes of Health website, with overview on asthma guidelines. http://www.nhlbi.nih.gov/guidelines/asthma/.

New York City Department of Health. (2001). *Asthma in New York City*. New York: Childhood Asthma Initiative.

Nicholas, S. W., et al. (2005). Addressing the childhood asthma crisis in Harlem: The Harlem Children's Zone asthma initiative. *American Journal of Public Health* 95, no. 2: 245–49.

Parker, E. A., et al. (2003). Community action against asthma: Examining the partnership process of a community-based participatory research project. *Journal of General Internal Medicine* 18, no. 7: 558–67.

Roxy to the Rescue (Adolescent Asthma). Educational video. Milner-Fenwick.

Stout, J. W., et al. (1998). The Asthma Outreach Project: A promising approach to comprehensive asthma management. *Journal of Asthma* 35, no. 1: 119–27.

Swider, S. M. (2002). Outcome effectiveness of community health workers: An integrative literature review. *Public Health Nursing* 19, no. 1: 11–20.

[5]

Start Right Coalition

Building on Community Initiatives for Childhood Immunization Promotion

SALLY E. FINDLEY WITH MARTHA SÁNCHEZ, MIRIAM MEJÍA, MARIO DRUMMONDS, and MATILDE IRIGOYEN

Although community-based partnerships of community and medical providers have been recommended for immunization, Start Right was one of the first to put into practice a truly community-driven childhood immunization coalition.

In 1989–91 northern Manhattan was one of the communities where the nationwide measles epidemic hit hard. In response, several community groups, led by Alianza Dominicana, joined the New York City Department of Health and Mental Hygiene to offer measles vaccinations at locations throughout the community. Over a thousand children were vaccinated in the space of a few days. While this mop-up action is what effectively halts a current outbreak, it does not include the kind of lasting, systemic changes needed to ward off future epidemics of measles—or other highly contagious childhood diseases such as varicella (chicken pox) or pertussis (whooping cough). The measles epidemic awakened the community to the problem of undervaccination. To be completely vaccinated requires repeated visits to the child's primary care physician from birth through age 18 months. Parents need to make the visits according to the recommended schedule, and medical providers need to make sure that they give all the required shots when children are seen. If all goes according to schedule, children will be completely vaccinated by age 19 months, a month after the last vaccinations are due; allowing for delays in getting the final vaccinations, national standards call for 90 percent vaccination rates for children 19–35 months of age.

86

Promoting Health and Primary Care

TABLE 5.1

Making a Difference: Start Right

PROBLEM: DISPARITIES IN CHILDHOOD IMMUNIZATION RATES (4:3:1:3)
NYC overall: 80%
Harlem: 47%
NMCVC coalition area: 63%

SOLUTION
Start Right, a bottom-up, community-driven approach to integrate immunization
  promotion activities within existing community programs

RESULTS
10,000 parents participated
Vaccination rates increased to 96. 8% (exceeded rate for New York City and
  United States, and Healthy People 2010 goal of 90%)

Sources: New York City Department of Health Survey (2000); surveys conducted by NMIP
(1999); National Health Statistics (2007).

Despite the scare of 1989–1991, in the mid-1990s the northern Manhattan vaccination rate was well below the national, if not the global, levels (table 5.1). Indeed, the community vaccination rates were at the same level as in Bamako, Mali, where I (Sally Findley) had participated in efforts to raise vaccination rates. The global expanded immunization program recently had been launched, so this seemed an opportune moment to bring the global lessons home to our community. The Northern Manhattan Start Right Coalition, whose aim was to decrease disparities in vaccination rates, grew out of our concern and the knowledge that we, like communities all over the world, could do something to raise vaccination rates. This chapter tells how the coalition was molded by the concerns of the community, supported by the Northern Manhattan Community Voices Initiative, and evolved through time into a strong academic-community partnership.

Evolution and Development of the Northern Manhattan
Start Right Coalition

In the years immediately after the measles epidemic, under the joint leadership of the New York City Department of Health and the Children's

Defense Fund, Children's Vaccination Program Networks were established. Networks were established in Harlem, under the leadership of Martha Sánchez at the Northern Manhattan Perinatal Partnership (NMPP), and in Washington Heights, under the leadership of Miriam Mejía at Alianza Dominicana. These networks, which predated the establishment of Northern Manhattan Community Voices Coalition, met monthly and collaborated in a number of immunization promotion events, such as health fairs or community leafleting. They produced community-appropriate flyers that were tailored to address the specific concerns of parents in our community; for example, one flyer addressed concerns in the African American community about childhood immunizations increasing HIV risk.

Paralleling these community coalitions, the pediatric provider networks serving northern Manhattan came together under Matilde Irigoyen's leadership to form the Northern Manhattan Immunization Partnership (NMIP). This network of fourteen clinics was established to make systematic changes in vaccination delivery practices, such as development of a networkwide immunization registry or a simplified vaccination flow sheet for clinical charts. With support from the National Immunization Program of the Centers for Disease Control (CDC), NMIP instituted regular chart reviews at all participating clinics to assess their own vaccination rates and then assist them in adopting practice improvements to raise their vaccination rates. At the same time, NMIP reached out to the community to learn from families about barriers they faced in having their children vaccinated.

With the launching of the NMCVC, there was a renewed commitment to improving health care for the community's families. I cochaired the Health Promotion and Disease Prevention working group, and, as part of the initial ascertainment of community health problems and priorities, we collected 482 individual surveys, conducted focus groups, dialogued with 13 community leaders, and completed numerous community health needs assessments. We administered surveys to 48 community providers, and the HP/DP working group collaborated with the New York City Department of Health and Mental Hygiene's Turning Point initiative to convene a community-wide dialogue in which 225 community residents participated. Finally, Community Voices convened a forum to review the findings from the exploration in order to select priority program areas. As reported in part 1 of this book, childhood immunization was one of the top priorities identified in these multiple channels of discovery. We found that the community had low rates of immunization coverage and that parents had problems keeping their children's vaccinations up-to-date.

Low Immunization Coverage Rates

Northern Manhattan lagged behind the rest of the city in protecting its children from the risk of infectious diseases. According to the 1998–99 National Immunization Survey, the citywide basic immunization coverage rate was 80 percent for children ages 19 to 35 months. The 1999 coverage surveys conducted by the NMIP at the eleven New York Presbyterian Hospital, Harlem Hospital, and St. Luke's-Roosevelt clinical practices showed that the northern Manhattan coverage rate for the basic immunization series (4:3:1:3 or 4 diphtheria-tetanus-pertussis [DTaP], 3 polio, 1 measles-mumps-rubella [MMR], and 3 Haemophilus influenza b [Hib] vaccinations) for children ages 19 to 35 months was only 47 percent, almost 30 percent less than the city average.

Keeping Children's Vaccinations Up-to-Date

The NMIP team conducted interviews with parents of children under age 3 throughout the community: at five clinics with 362 parents, two pediatric emergency departments with 432 parents, and the five Special Supplemental Nutrition Program for Women, Infants and Children sites with 220 parents. Regardless of where the families were interviewed, these surveys confirmed the low immunization coverage rates observed at the practices. They also provided insights into some of the situations that make it difficult for parents to keep their children's vaccinations up to date. We found that:

1. *Children were not up-to-date with immunizations:* Only half the children (49%) were current or up-to-date with their immunizations. Further, 82 percent of the parents whose children were not up-to-date mistakenly thought that they were current with all vaccinations.

2. *Families had problems with insurance:* Parents said they had difficulties maintaining health insurance coverage for their children,

with 25 percent having gaps in coverage in the first year of life, and 23 percent of the children uninsured at the time of the interview.

Detailed analyses of the data from these surveys showed that there were health care correlates of the children's immunization status. Children without health insurance coverage at birth were more likely to be behind in vaccinations (47 percent current with immunizations among those with insurance at birth versus 31 percent for those without insurance at birth). Children who started their immunizations late also were less likely to be current with immunizations.

To learn more about the difficulties of obtaining immunizations, we conducted four focus groups in Spanish and English, at both clinical and community organizations. The focus groups revealed that:

- Parents believed in vaccinations and wanted their children to have them.
- Parents did not always know what the immunizations were for or when they were due for their child.
- Some parents were unsure about where to go to find out what their child needed.
- Parents wanted reminders from their doctor about immunizations and more opportunities to ask questions about immunizations during office visits.
- Parents encountered problems taking time off to get to the clinic.

The following statement from one mother summarizes the sentiment that parents did not understand immunizations or their significance: "The new mothers just sit there and take the appointment, and don't realize that it's important for their child to go once a month to get their shot and why. They don't know why they're really taking them to the doctor, how many shots they're getting, stuff like that."

Based on these findings, we concluded that there was much work for the coalition in closing the gap. Further, our investigations pointed to several things we could do that would help parents in the community make sure their children were vaccinated on time:

1. Create more opportunities to learn about immunizations, from the community and from the medical providers.

2. Provide more information about immunization logistics, both when and where to get them, including reminders.
3. Provide assistance in obtaining and maintaining health insurance.
4. Give more feedback to physicians on how well they were doing as well as tips on how they could ensure that their practice routine was proactive in delivering all immunizations on time.

These recommendations were consistent with national guidelines for ensuring immunization coverage. Given the congruence in assessments of what needed to be done, the coalition proceeded to develop a program to promote immunizations incorporating these basic objectives.

When the CDC included reduction of childhood immunization disparities in its original Reach 2010 call for proposals, we were ready. We convened a joint meeting of the Harlem and Washington Heights Childhood Vaccination Program Networks and the NMIP. At that historic meeting, we decided to merge these three coalitions into the Northern Manhattan Start Right Coalition, which included all the organizations that had participated in child immunization activities with the Children's Vaccination Program Networks, the clinical networks of the NMIP, and the Mailman School of Public Health, one of the leading partners in both the NMCVC and NMIP and my home base. During a several month process we explored alternatives for the combined coalition. With many contributions from the coalition members, I prepared a proposal on behalf of the coalition to the Reach 2010 program.

We adopted the ambitious goal of eliminating the disparity in the childhood immunization rate for children in the community, with the objective of increasing the immunization coverage rate to 90 percent for the vaccinations due before age 3. We established a target of enrolling ten thousand children under age 3, focusing on the children who have the greatest difficulty achieving on-time immunizations, namely, those with no or interrupted insurance, those who had started late or missed immunizations in the middle of the series, and those who had not stayed connected to their primary care provider. Start Right became one of only three coalitions out of twenty-three funded by the Reach 2010 program to implement community-based strategies to eliminate racial and ethnic health disparities in childhood immunizations. I invited Martha Sánchez to join me at Columbia in leading the coalition's efforts, and she moved from NMPP to Columbia to serve as the overall coalition coordinator.

The initial year of the coalition's support was devoted to preparing a community action plan for eliminating programs to reduce the community's immunization disparity. We asked all organizations to identify the programs that had *and* had not worked to promote immunization coverage gains. We collectively reviewed the lessons learned and identified the following main strategies:

- The most effective strategies for promoting immunizations in the community had been activities that engaged families one-on-one.
- We wanted to build on what we were already doing well with parents, community development and social service programs. Rather than trying to add yet another program to the already complicated mix of activities juggled by families with young children, we decided to incorporate immunization promotion into their ongoing programs.
- We needed a partnership with the medical providers, to make sure that all children received their vaccinations on time. Our view was to work from both sides: to enable families to be more proactive in seeking immunizations and to facilitate more timely and complete vaccination delivery.

After months of deliberation, we agreed on the following six guiding principles for our coalition's program: community decision making and leadership; integration with community social service programs; community health workers as peer educators; parental empowerment through education, reminders, and social support; evidence-based immunization promotion activities; and linkages with health providers to promote provider best-practices. The remainder of this chapter describes how these guiding principles were integrated into the coalition's program and contributed to the success of the coalition in attaining its goals.

Start Right Coalition in Action: Turning Guiding Principles into Program

We adopted a model of health promotion from within, namely, integration of immunization promotion activities within existing community programs, organized in accord with the six guiding principles consistent with community-based participatory action research, as follows.

Community Decision Making and Leadership

Consistent with the Community Voices framework, we established a shared leadership structure. Decisions were made by consensus at monthly meetings, held in rotation at each member organization. The coalition included twenty-three community organizations: five community social service organizations, eight child-care providers, two housing advocacy organizations, three WIC programs, three primary care provider networks, one city agency, and one academic partner. Leadership was shared between the academic and community partners, with two lead community organizations responsible for oversight of activities for the members in their respective neighborhoods, Washington Heights/Inwood or Harlem. Educational materials and reminder cards were developed by the coalition as a whole, produced centrally, and then distributed throughout the membership. Adhering to recommendations for community partners to establish their own targets, each member identified the programs into which Start Right would be integrated, the number of families to be enrolled, and the additional support needed to accomplish these goals. Subcontracts ensured that each member had funds to pay staff for the additional work required as well as funds for incentives and other supplies needed to implement the program. Accountability was maintained through monthly activity reports to the hub leaders, consistent with recommendations for shared accountability among partners.

We met monthly to discuss our activities, highlighting successes and the creative solutions to problems. In this way, good ideas developed by one organization were spread to other members. Examples of this spread of good ideas included a simplified tracking form for keeping track of vaccinations children had received and reminders parents needed; the coalition vaccination information pamphlet; and practical reminder "ticklers" generated from the coalition database. Conversely, if members encountered problems enrolling or working with families, they could ask others for advice and assistance.

Integration into Community Programs

Growing out of the Community Voices process and informed by our personal passions for community empowerment, we saw the primary home for our program as the many community programs making up the coalition. We therefore chose to integrate immunization promotion activities into existing community programs, as recommended for effective community health promotion programs. Applying the principle of asset-based programming, we developed the coalition program around the strategy of building capacity to provide information and assistance about immunizations within our already strong programs for families with young children.

We identified six categories of programs where immunization could be incorporated into routine activities: parenting guidance and assistance, child care, facilitated enrollment for health insurance, the Special Supplemental Nutrition Program for Women, Infants and Children, housing assistance, and referrals from primary care clinics. We developed a practical implementation guide to help program staff tailor their activities to include immunization promotion: how and when to identify eligible parents, enroll them, and give immunization reminders. Organizations could implement the coalition program at one or more of their programs. Our evaluation component was approved by the Columbia University Medical Center Institutional Review Board.

Community Health Workers as Peer Educators

We chose to use peer educators or community health workers as the prime agents of change. This was consistent with recommendations regarding effective communications to promote immunizations or other health behaviors, particularly those with large immigrant populations such as in our community. Each organization specified the number of community health workers they would train, generally selecting individuals who could add immunization promotion to their duties for existing programs at the organization. Several multiservice organizations trained all their staff so they could identify and refer candidates for immunization promotion activities.

We at Mailman School of Public Health (myself and Martha Sánchez) developed a five-part training curriculum, which we offered with assistance from the Bureau of Immunization of the New York City Department of Health and Mental Hygiene and the hub leaders, particularly Miriam Mejía at Alianza Dominicana. All trainees received training in using immunization education materials with families so they could be prepared for a wide range of questions and concerns. The training included the implementation guidelines for fitting the immunization promotion activities into the routine program activities. Those community health workers who would be enrolling families were trained and certified in Good Clinical Practices through the Columbia University Medical Center Institutional Review Board.

Between 2000 and 2007 the coalition trained 998 community health workers. We assessed their improvement in understanding immunizations (which diseases, how immunizations work, why repeat vaccination doses are needed) using pre- and posttests. For the 516 who completed such tests, the average increase in immunization competency was 14 percent, from 82 percent to 96 percent. At any given time, between 150 and 200 of those trained remained active, with the remainder leaving their agency or being promoted to other jobs. Most (98%) were women, primarily Latina and African American, and residents in the community; many were bilingual. These women were highly motivated to give back to the community.

We received annual feedback from 175 community health workers about their work and the adequacy of their training. It was universally enthusiastic and positive. Box 5.1 provides examples of their comments.

BOX 5.1
Community Health Workers Feedback

"I have learned a lot doing this kind of work. Before I didn't know how to read cards. I learned about coalitions."

"It helps me keep on helping the community. Many parents are not aware of the importance of vaccinations."

"This helped me to understand things I did not know before. The information is good for informing parents. I learned how to use the calendar to make parents ready for appointments."

"Learning how to read the immunization card was one of the best trainings I've ever gotten, because now I can tell parents if their children are up-to-date or not."

"Now, when moms go to the doctor they know what is going on and understand what he tells them. So they come back and thank us for helping them understand."

The following is an account by one of the Start Right community health workers who work in the context of a parenting program in the nearby public housing development. She said:

> I do outreach in the St. Nicholas Houses; that's a NYC Housing Authority project. I go door-to-door. If they are at home and answer, we discuss immunizations with them; for those not home, we put the flyer under the door. I often get calls back from parents asking what the flyer is about, and then I explain to them. I try to bring them into our office [down the block] to discuss immunizations and especially the importance of getting immunizations on time. Often after we have talked and looked at the literature, they can answer their own questions. And if not, they are better prepared to go and talk to the doctors.
>
> Our most effective work is through the activities and events that we do. We know that toddlers like to have fun and parents need things to do with their kids. We do a toddler jamboree, where kids 0–3 are invited. While the toddlers are having fun, we talk with the parents about immunizations and make sure that they are informed. Then we check their cards to see if they are up-to-date. If they are not, we work to get them up-to-date so that their kids are ready for school.

This account demonstrates how immunization promotion was integrated into the ongoing activities of the organization. We were not organizing immunization events; we organized fun, educational events for the parents and their children and added immunization promotion to those events. In this way, each organization kept the doors open for the multiple interactions needed to help the parent through the entire immunization series with its five-plus visits to the doctor.

Parent Empowerment

To ensure that we reached families who did not have a regular doctor, most outreach was conducted within the thirty-two programs offered by our members, with additional outreach on a rotating schedule to WIC program sites and neighborhood pediatric providers. When eligible parents were identified, the trained coalition community health workers explained the program, invited them to participate, and asked for informed consent. Almost all (97%) chose to participate, with only 3 percent refusals. Between October 2000 and May 2007 we enrolled 10,251 parents of children under age 5, exceeding our enrollment target of 10,000 children. The most common recruitment programs were WIC (26% of children); facilitated enrollment for health insurance (20%); child care/Head Start, including family day-care provider networks (20%); parenting programs, including home visiting programs (19%); housing/tenant advocacy programs (9%); and community primary care practices or welfare offices (9%) (see fig. 5.1)

Each year parents were asked what they liked the most and the least about the program, and box 5.2 is a sampling of what they liked most.

Because our immunization promotion activities were integrated into programs vital to the families, such as their children's child-care program or getting health insurance, parents could easily understand that the program was for their children's health, not just the problem of immunizations. This structural context of organizational caring was reinforced by the community health workers' empathy. In the words of one participant: "I liked everything, especially when you see how much they care for the kids' health. She showed me she cared what happens to my child."

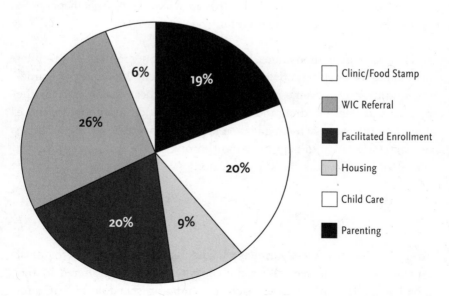

Figure 5.1 Enrollment into Start Right by Programmatic Strategy (October 2000–March 2007)

BOX 5.2
What Parents Liked Most

Importance of immunizations

"I like the information we got about the diseases you get when the children don't get vaccinated."

"The program made me more aware about my child's immunization and how important it is to have them done on time."

"This program educates the parents. I did not know about children's vaccines. Because of the program, I realized my child needed more shots."

"My child has some of his shots, but the program helped me to make and keep appointments for the rest of my child's shots. I think the program did all that they could. The rest is up to me."

"I learned to read my child's immunization card. I realized that my child needed a vaccine."

"They broke down the information so that it was easier to understand."

Parent empowerment

"It helped me by giving me information on places to go for shots, and also handing out lots of materials on vaccinations."

"I learned how to inquire about the vaccinations my baby should get."

"I asked my doctor more. I had been anxious that the vaccine has viruses. I felt that giving the virus would be harmful. The doctor told me that it was okay because you get immune to it."

Networking and social support

"They told me about resources available to people like me that I didn't know about. I have passed on this information to other people about vaccines."

"They put me in touch with other women and we shared opinions. That helped me to get stronger and be more independent and got my mind positive before it became negative."

"I would say that this is a place for moms where you can educate yourself about your children and meet other moms like you. They can benefit from the program when they work together."

Evidence-Based Immunization Promotion Activities

Our immunization promotion activities incorporated activities identified as the most effective, evidence-based strategies. These included community-based immunization education; reminders of upcoming immunizations and recalls for missed immunizations; and provider feedback and other techniques to reduce missed opportunities for immunizations when the child visits the primary care provider.

We developed our own bilingual informational package, from which each community health worker selected materials to address participants' concerns or fears about immunizations, such as whether vaccinations would hurt their babies or could spread HIV/AIDS. The most commonly used item was our own brochure with pictorial and factual information about the diseases and the city's schedule for immunizations required for school enrollment. Community health workers were trained to elicit parental concerns and use the materials to help parents address their fears and learn the facts about immunizations. They used the coalition brochure to explain the dangers of each disease and emphasized the parents' role in protecting their children from the dangerous diseases portrayed in the brochure. The community health workers also were trained in how to role-play conversations with the children's medical providers, sharing their own experiences and anxieties with the parents, giving them space for expression of fears and doubts. Finally, the workers gave parents written reminders for their next vaccinations.

After the initial educational interactions, the reminders were the core of the intervention. Community health workers followed up with personalized reminders two weeks in advance of the next shot due date, and afterward to make sure the child received the shots. The reminders took many forms: birthday cards, text messages, notes sent home with the children from day care, discussions during home visits, special letters or postcards, telephone calls, and reminders added into the routine follow-up for the parents' primary program. Parents interacted with their community health workers an average of 5.1 times, with an average of 2.1 reminders or recalls per child. These interactions were in the context of each organization's ongoing program activities. For example, at the child-care programs, reminders were given directly to each parent by the child-care staff, while at parenting programs they were given during a home visit or meeting with staff.

The last evidence-based program component included activities to prevent missed opportunities, namely, when a child is seen by the primary care provider but is not given any or all needed immunizations. We encouraged participants to take their coalition-generated vaccination reminders with them to doctor's visits and request vaccinations for their child. We helped the parents advocate for receiving all vaccinations for which a child was due, and not to accept being told to come back to receive some of them at a second, and billable, visit.

Linkages to Health Care Providers

The coalition helped parents maintain connections to their primary care providers; for example, by making appointments or escorting parents to appointments. At the same time, coalition staff maintained direct connections with the primary care providers, inviting families seen at the clinics to participate in the coalition.

Under the leadership of Matilde Irigoyen, head of the General Pediatrics Group Practice of New York Presbyterian Hospital and director of the Pediatrics Fellowship program at Columbia University, the coalition promoted best practices for tracking immunizations at provider sites through use of immunization registries—a very important step in this community where many children are seen by two or more medical providers. She was instrumental in launching the hospital immunization registry and creating linkages between the hospital and city immunization registries, allowing providers to accurately assess immunization status using web-based software in their offices. Nonetheless, many vaccinations were not reported to the registry, with 29–42% of vaccinations recorded on the children's cards missing from these registries. Therefore, we established a data warehouse integrating information from the child's vaccination card with records from the major hospital registry serving children in Washington Heights/ Inwood and the New York City Immunization Registry. This complete accounting of all vaccinations was critical to maintaining accurate reminders and recalls to families. Without the data warehouse we would not have complete vaccination information, which is needed to compare to the National Immunization Survey, which includes all vaccinations recorded on the child's vaccination card. In addition, the coalition database had features designed by the coalition to flag children needing reminders or follow-up, as well as an alert when the child had completed all immunizations and was due a thank you gift.

The coalition database was decentralized so that each organization was responsible for entry to and updating of the records of children whom they had enrolled into the program. We did monthly data exchanges to update the partner and main coalition databases. By 2007 the coalition database had records for the 10,251 enrolled children and included more than 185,000 shots.

Coalition Outcomes: Elimination of the Immunization Disparity

Participation and Study Group

Between October 2000 and May 2007 the coalition reached out to 31,156 parents, screened 11,749 parents for eligibility, found 10,539 eligible children, and enrolled 10,251. Across all years, the refusal rate was 3 percent. Each year 5.3 percent of the children were lost to follow-up, primarily due to moving out of the area or a change in phone number. Because the national comparison group includes only children 19–35 months of age, we restricted the sample in this report to 6,990 children aged 19–35 months on April 1 of each year, 2002–2007.

Measures

We assessed vaccination coverage as the percentage of children aged 19–35 months as of April 1 of the estimate year who had completed all the vaccinations for the complete vaccination series (4:3:1:3:3), as recommended by the Advisory Committee on Immunization Practices. We compared our rates with those published for the same age-group for children in New York City and the total United States, as published in table 29 of the appropriate year from the National Immunization Survey. We determined if our rates were significantly different from the city or national rates using the National Immunization Survey 95 percent confidence intervals.

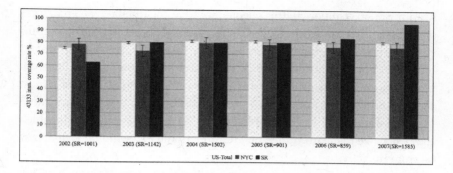

Figure 5.2   Coalition versus National and New York City Immunization
Coverage Rates by Race/Ethnicity, 2000—2007*
*(Children 19–35 months of age as of April 1 of estimate year)
Note: National and NYC estimates from National Immunization Survey, Jan.–Dec. for
the reported year, except 2007, which is Jan.–June only; Table 29 (Race and Ethnicity
by State and IAP). 95% CI inverval shown in braces for U.S. and NYC estimates.

Vaccination Coverage Rate Disparities

As shown in figure 5.2, in 2002 the coalition's average vaccination coverage rate of 63 percent (shown in black) was significantly below the national
and city vaccination coverage rates. From 2002 to 2005 the coalition's vaccination coverage rate of 80 percent was no longer significantly different
from the New York City or national averages. In 2006 the coalition's vaccination rate increased to 84.1 percent, still within the confidence interval
for the city rate, but significantly exceeding the national rates for the total
national population. In 2007, when we redoubled its follow-up efforts, the
coalition's rate increased again, to 96.8 percent, surpassing the city rate, as
well as the national rate. While the U.S. immunization rate had not yet
reached the Healthy People 2010 goal of 90 percent for childhood immunization coverage, the coalition's rates exceeded that goal.

Discussion

Although community-based partnerships of community and medical providers have been recommended for immunization promotion, our coalition
was one of the first to put into practice a truly community-driven childhood

immunization coalition. In this chapter, we have documented the guidelines and procedures by which we developed and implemented our vision for eliminating childhood immunization disparities. The careful planning to build the capacity of the community to mobilize parents and facilitate on-time immunizations paid off at many levels. We created a cadre of almost a thousand community health workers who incorporated immunization promotion into their work, regardless of the goals of the program in which they work. We made immunization reminders and follow-ups a normal part of program activities.

Most important, we changed the nature of the conversation between parents and doctors about immunizations. With our support and reminders, parents no longer passively received information and appointment cards for immunizations. Those who had never understood or were afraid of immunizations had their questions and fears addressed and could raise further questions with their providers. When the provider failed to initiate the vaccination process at a visit, the parent could request immunizations, making sure that this was not a missed opportunity for the parent.

Our bottom-up, community-driven approach proved quite successful. More than ten thousand parents participated in the program, and by the third year of operation the coalition had eliminated immunization disparities for children whose parents participated in the program. The children's vaccination coverage rates matched or exceeded the rates for children in New York City and nationwide, and in 2007 we exceeded the Healthy People 2010 goal of 90 percent.

The road to these achievements included some difficult patches, where we had to change course in order to achieve our goals. The most difficult challenge was the reduced access to immunization records associated with the passage of the Health Insurance Portability and Accountability Act of 1996 (HIPAA) Privacy Rule regulations. When we originally planned the program, we anticipated that our community health workers would at least be able to view their enrollees' immunization registry records, as was agreed in the consent form. However, city and hospital regulations did not permit access except through the child's health care provider. Nor were our community health workers able to update the registry if they found that the child's recent vaccinations had not been reported. This meant that we had to develop our own parallel database, which not only added time and expense to the program but also made it more difficult for the community health workers to know when the children actually received their vaccinations. In the future we recommend that registries be designed to allow community-based CHW access, at least in read-only format, so that they can be most timely in their reminders to parents. Our experience shows that this is completely within the range of capacity for community health workers, as demonstrated by the number of workers in our program who became adept at using the database.

Another huge frustration was the fact that even with mandatory reporting, many children's vaccinations were not reported to the city Immunization Registry. This also required additional follow-up with parents, who would otherwise not have to bring their children's vaccination cards for review by the CHW. As the registry has matured, reporting has increased, but efforts still need to be redoubled to encourage complete and timely reporting by all health care providers.

Our experience demonstrates the power of the Community Voices approach to working within the community to promote change. We believe that four design features were key to our success. First, we sought out families throughout the community, regardless of connection to a medical provider or even the presence of health insurance. Thus, we reached the highest-risk parents who would have been excluded from provider-based interventions, namely, the low-income, minority, and, often, immigrant parents who did not have a regular medical home for their children's care. Second, our community health workers were trusted faces and voices in the community. Through the frank conversations possible with CHWs, parents could discuss their fears or concerns, knowing they would be understood and respected. With the ongoing support from the CHWs, parents were motivated to make immunization promotion one of their essential parenting responsibilities. This normative shift laid the foundation for the improved communication with doctors reported by parents in their feedback to the coalition. Third, our community-based approach to providing reminders to parents guaranteed not only their delivery but also their culturally appropriate context. The parents received the reminders from the program staff they saw regularly and trusted, leaving no doubt that the reminder was "really" meant for them. Lastly, the immunization promotion activities were integrated directly into routine community development, social service, and educational programs, so that immunization promotion complemented rather than competed with the other critical services families were already obtaining. By linking immunization promotion to other priority activities, we made it possible for the parents to meet two needs at once: their children's health and other basic needs. We believe that these key features can be applied to other problems and are a part of the lessons from Community Voices: broad community outreach, peers or CHWs as the main communicators and motivators, community-based reminders and information, and integration of health promotion into ongoing community programs.

References

Barnes, K., S. M. Friedman, P. B. Namerow, and J. Honig (1999). Impact of community volunteers on immunization rates of children younger than 2 years. *Archives of Pediatrics and Adolescent Medicine* 153: 518–24.

Briss, P. A., et al. (2000). Reviews of evidence regarding interventions to improve vaccination coverage in children, adolescents, and adults. The Task Force on Community Preventive Services. *American Journal of Preventive Medicine* 18: 97–140.

Crawford, N. W., and J. P. Buttery (2008). Minimizing missed opportunities to vaccinate. *Journal of Paediatrics and Child Health* 44, no. 6: 315–16.

Findley, S., M. Irigoyen, M. Sanchez, L. Guzman, et al. (2006). Community-based strategies to promote childhood immunizations. *Health Promotion Practice* 7 (Suppl. 3): 191S–200S.

Findley, S., M. Irigoyen, M. Sanchez, M. Stockwell, et al. (2008). Effectiveness of a community coalition for improving child vaccination rates in New York City. *American Journal of Public Health* 98: 1959–62.

Institute of Medicine of the National Academies. (2003). *Speaking of health: Assessing health communication strategies for diverse populations.* Washington, D.C.: National Academies Press.

Israel, B. A., et al. (2003). Critical issues in developing and following community based participatory research principles. In *Community-based participatory research for health*, ed. M. Minkler and N. Wallerstein, 53–76. San Francisco: Jossey-Bass.

Jacobson, V., and P. Szilagyi, P. (2005). Patient reminder and patient recall systems to improve immunization rates. *Cochrane Database Systems Review* 3, CD003941.

LeBaron, C. W., et al. (1998). The impact of interventions by a community-based organization on inner-city vaccination coverage. Fulton County, Georgia, 1992–1993. *Archives of Pediatrrics and Adolescent Medicine* 152, no. 4: 327–32.

Minkler, M., and T. Hancock (2003). Community-driven asset identification and issue selection. In *Community-based participatory research for health*, ed. M. Minkler and N. Wallerstein. San Francisco: Jossey-Bass.

Rickert, D .L., A. M. Shefer, and L. E. Rodewald (2003). Counting the shots: A model for immunization screening and referral in nonmedical settings. *Pediatrics* 111: 1297–1302.

Ringel, M. (1998). Practical solutions to boost adult and childhood immunization rates. *Medical Management Network* 6, no. 3: 1–5.

Rizzo, C. (2006). Linking practices with community programs to improve immunization rates. *Pediatric Annals* 35, no. 7: 513–15.

Szilagyi, P., and L. Rodewald (1996). Missed opportunities for immunizations: A review of the evidence. *Journal of Public Health Management and Practice* 2, no. 1: 18–25.

Selected Additional References

Centers for Disease Control (1991). Summary of notifiable diseases, United States. 1990. *MMWR Morbidity Mortality Weekly Report*, Oct. 4, 39, no. 53: 1–61 (for the 1989–1991 measles outbreak in the United States and various surveillance data).

—— (2009). Advisory Committee on Immunization Practices. http://www.needle tips.org/acip/ (for vaccine recommendations for newborns/infants).

Findley, S., et al. (2003). Community-provider partnerships to reduce immunization disparities: Field report from northern Manhattan. *American Journal of Public Health* 93, no. 71: 1041–44 (for data collected for the vaccination efforts in northern Manhattan).

Immunization Action Coalition (2009). "Summary of Recommendations for Childhood and Adolescent Immunization." http://www.immunize.org/catg.d/ p2010.pdf (for vaccine recommendations for newborns/infants).

Northern Manhattan Start Right Coalition. "Directory of Immunization Coalitions: A Project of the Immunization Action Coalition." http://www.izcoalitions .org/search/OrgShow.asp?OID=OID260.

U.S. Department of Health and Human Services (1996). "The Health Insurance Portability and Accountability Act of 1996 (HIPAA) Privacy Rule." http://www .hhs.gov/ocr/privacy/ (for limits that community health workers have around accessing medical records).

[6]

The Legacy Smoking-Cessation Project

CHERYL RAGONESI, MARTIN OVALLES, and DANIEL F. SEIDMAN

> They say that time changes things, but you actually have to change them yourself.
>
> —Andy Warhol

About six months into the first year of the national Community Voices project, the American Legacy Foundation became interested in collaborating with the W. K. Kellogg Foundation on smoking prevention/cessation programs. The Legacy Foundation was relatively new and had been established as an outcome of the "tobacco settlement," which required the tobacco companies to fund an independent foundation to counter smoking. At the time, Legacy was particularly interested in reaching individuals in low-income communities and communities of color, who were targets for intense advertisement by the tobacco companies (see box 6.1).

Legacy's president met with the senior program officer at the Kellogg Foundation to discuss a collaboration in which all of the thirteen funded Community Voices sites would become eligible to apply for a supplemental American Legacy Foundation grant. The grant was to be used to plan and implement tobacco cessation/prevention programs for the underserved communities in which they were working. According to Allan Formicola, who helped to arrange the collaboration, "This was a perfect opportunity for both foundations. Legacy wanted to reach out to low-income neighborhoods where there were, as they perceived, targeted campaigns on smoking, especially to children. And the Community Voices sites were working in many of those communities throughout the nation." All sites were invited to apply for four-year grants of $200,000. Eight of the thirteen sites received grants, and the Northern Manhattan Community Voices Collaborative was one of them.

NMCVC was able to draw upon several strengths for the program it was funded to implement. The first strength was that Columbia University Medical Center had a nationally known expert in tobacco cessation, Dan Seidman. In particular, he had developed a smoking cessation program at the College of Dental Medicine, which was established in 1996. At that time, there were not as yet all of the resources for smoking cessation/prevention programs that have now become available through the New York City Health Department. The cessation program at the College of Dental Medicine was the only one in northern Manhattan, and the only one operating within the Columbia University Medical Center and New York Presbyterian Hospital. It operated only one day a week to care for all those for whom it was imperative to quit smoking because they were diagnosed with smoking-related diseases, as well as for those who wanted to quit as a way to better health. To make cessation more easily available to the population, the NMCVC proposal envisioned using that program as a model for developing similar cessation programs in several of the primary care facilities of New York Presbyterian Hospital and other such health centers operating in northern Manhattan.

The second strength was that NMCVC partner Alianza Dominicana already had much experience in developing and working with youth. Under the NMCVC umbrella and Dan Seidman's leadership, a team that included a social worker, Cheryl Ragonesi, and a translator/community health worker, Martin Ovalles, was brought together to implement the project.

In this chapter, the three of us on the team collectively describe the project and its goals and strategies and provide a summary of its overall achievements. We then focus on a selection of programs using our own voices and those of the patients who were served and whose lives were transformed.

BOX 6.1
Special Targets: Youth

Age at which adolescents and preadolescents who smoke start in Washington Heights[1]

11–13

Youth heavy daily smokers in Washington Heights[1]
Female: 55%
Male: 35%

Ratio of antismoking messages to tobacco ads around schools in Latino neighborhoods [1]

1:11

Increase in Hispanic youth smoking rates from 1989 to 1997[2]

20%

[1]Alianza Dominicana (1995).
[2]U.S. Department of Health and Human Services (1999).

Project Description

The Community Voices–Legacy Smoking Cessation project was designed to increase community awareness of the effects of tobacco use through clinical patient services, education, and outreach. The goals of the program were threefold: (1) to increase access to smoking cessation services to minority populations in northern Manhattan, (2) to prevent onset of tobacco use by adolescents through increased outreach and education efforts, and (3) to develop programs that target smoking cessation among minority youth and families. To meet these goals, the NMCVC implemented a two-tiered program composed of smoking cessation services for adults in a variety of clinical settings and a community-based youth led mini-grant initiative.

The Northern Manhattan Community Voices–Legacy program achieved significant outcomes and sustainable policy changes. The smoking cessation program established a strong foundation and infrastructure to offer clinical community-based cessation services and strengthen community capacity to counteract the tobacco industry marketing campaigns targeting youth. Through the efforts of the Community Voices–Legacy program, there are now more effective community-based smoking cessation services available in northern Manhattan. The model program, established at the clinic of Columbia University's College of Dental Medicine, has also been replicated at the Thelma C. Davidson Adair Medical/Dental Center and at various sites at New York Presbyterian Hospital.

The project employed innovative methods within its programs. For example, to ensure sustainability and promote the expansion of services at other sites, the Community Voices–Legacy program offered continuing education seminars for providers at multiple community health centers. Practitioners from many disciplines, including physicians, dentists, nurses, social workers, and medical/dental assistants at Columbia University and New York Presbyterian Hospital, have participated in these educational seminars. Over the course of the years, we have trained approximately three hundred practitioners in smoking cessation.

To meet the needs of our communities, which are predominantly Dominican and African American, we knew it was essential that culturally appropriate outreach was conducted, and that services remain sensitive to the challenges and strengths of the people living here. Furthermore, the residents of the community had relatively low incomes, and many were without health insurance coverage. To effectively address this underlying reality, the Community Voices–Legacy program instituted the community health worker model as part of two main components (Youth Initiative and Clinical Services). NMCVC also partnered with one of the largest social service organizations in the community, Alianza Dominicana, a community-based organization in Washington Heights. (For more information about the NMCVC community health worker program, see chapter 3.)

Another unique approach was the provision of mini-grants for youth in the community. In March 2002 Community Voices and Alianza Dominicana launched the Youth Tobacco Mini-Grant Initiative. The purpose of these mini-grants was to promote the creation and implementation of youth-led activities that aim to dissuade their peers from tobacco use in central Harlem and Washington Heights/Inwood. In June 2002 Community Voices funded twelve youth mini-grants projects. The projects typically incorporated art, drama, sports, media, music, and technology with a smoking cessation message. The funding was given to community-based organizations, faith-based organizations, and schools in Washington Heights/Inwood and Harlem. Approximately seventy youth participated in the initial round of funding.

In June 2003 we launched the second round of funding and did much of the same as we did in the first round. However, we gave mini-grants to new community-based organizations, faith-based organizations, and schools. Our goal was to expand the number of mini-grants given, as well as to extend the opportunity to be part of this endeavor to as many youth in the community as possible. We did give a few grants to some groups who had received grants in the first year. However, these were only given to organizations that proved that the expansion of their project would cast a larger net of awareness of the ill effects of tobacco in their communities. Overall eighteen youth organizations were funded in the second year.

In June 2004 the final round of youth-led antismoking campaigns was launched. Our main goal was to fund projects that we thought would be sustainable. To do this we picked fewer projects and provided them with the funds and support they would need to successfully carry out their projects and incorporate them into the fabric of their organizations for years to come. For example, a school in Harlem created beautiful banners with antismoking messages that we hope still hang on the walls at that school to this day. As a result of these grants, age-appropriate and culturally responsive projects were created and implemented and have become an established part of their host organizations. The youth groups also made plans to continue sharing the antismoking message with their larger community. This program has tremendously strengthened the leadership capacity of youth across the Harlem and Washington Heights communities. During a three-year time span from 2002 to 2004, more than two hundred youth participated in peer-led smoking-prevention projects, and hundreds more have heard the message about the dangers of smoking.

Since the initiation of the Community Voices–Legacy program, several community-based cessation services have also been established and formally integrated into the existing health delivery system of northern Manhattan. The participation and eventual institutional buy-in of New York Presbyterian Hospital, one of the community's largest health care providers, ensured the success and sustainability of the cessation services. Although the initial challenges and barriers were numerous, the outcome has proved to be worthwhile. Because of the Community Voices–Legacy program, northern Manhattan has an established institutional and community-based infrastructure to expand, replicate, and sustain the cessation efforts. Evidence of this is the successful implementation of the New York State Department of Health's Mailman School of Public Health Manhattan Tobacco Cessation Network. The efforts of this program, which were dedicated to reducing tobacco use through evidence-based smoking cessation treatment, were built on the success of the Community Voices–Legacy Smoking Cessation program.

Many lives have been deeply affected by this program. From the project staff, to the youth leaders, to the clients we served at the clinic, the program has had a life-changing effect that will continue to benefit the northern Manhattan community. The patient stories in two case studies vividly demonstrate the effectiveness of this program. The stories have been written by clients who successfully quit smoking and are verbatim. Both clients were interviewed by WNBC in the wake of the death of Peter Jennings, the news anchor who died of lung cancer and was a smoker for many years.

R.D.'S TOBACCO-CESSATION STORY

My reason for attending the smoke-enders clinic was simply to stop the damage smoking was doing to my teeth. After a dental exam, the dentist said if I do not stop smoking, I would possibly lose all of my teeth within a 2 year period. At this point in my life, I had been smoking cigarettes for 40 years.

I started smoking when I was 12 years old. I remember liking the effect cigarette smoke had on me right with the first cigarette. It had a calming effect and made my constant low-level anxiety disappear, temporarily. After about an hour, it would return. It did not take me long to connect the cigarette with the disappearance of the anxiety. Soon, I was smoking about 1 pack of cigarettes a day.

At age 16, I decided to quit and managed to do so on my own. But, after about 4 months, I suddenly had an overwhelming urge to smoke and gave in. I smoked a whole pack of cigarettes that day and have been smoking every day since. About every 2 to 3 years I try to quit smoking. It usually fails after about 24 hours; sometimes sooner.

(Continued)

The extent of my smoking can be roughly summarized as follows: Age 12 to 17: 1 pack/day; 17 to 19: 2 packs/day; 19 to 22: 3 packs/day; 22 to 31: 2 packs/day; 31 to 42: 1.5 packs/day; 42 to 52: 1 pack/day.

The dental clinic put me in touch with the smoke-enders clinic in December of 2004. They consist of a Clinical Psychologist, a Social Worker and a patient/clinic Coordinator. They also have access to medical and dental personnel for assistance, if needed. The clinic put a simple but effective plan in place for me. Their plan deals with the chemical dependence and the emotional/psychological dependence as two separate issues comprising the cigarette addiction. The chemical addiction is dealt with using the Nicoderm patch to minimize nicotine craving along with the Nicotrol Inhaler for handling momentary spikes in daily tension and anxiety. The emotional/psychological issues associated with cigarette addiction are dealt with in weekly 45-minute meetings with the Social Worker and Clinical Psychologist.

I quit smoking for the last time January 3, 2005, at 10 a.m. With the help of this clinic I have been smoke-free now for almost 8 months. In about 5 weeks, I will no longer be wearing the Nicoderm Patch. The Nicoderm Patch comes in 3 nicotine strengths; 21 mg, 14 mg and 7 mg. You start with the highest strength and every 3 months step down to the next lower strength patch. I am currently about 7 weeks with the lowest strength patch. The Nicotrol Inhaler works for me as I imagine "worry beads" work for an individual. Just holding the Inhaler calms me down. If I use the Inhaler, its ability to calm me occurs in just a few seconds. The literature accompanying the Inhaler says the device delivers nicotine to the brain in 15 to 20 minutes after inhaling. Obviously, there is a significant psychological component in its calming effect upon me.

If I have learned one thing from attending this clinic, it is that everything takes time to change. It takes time for old habits to permanently cease. It takes time for new habits to develop and become real. I have had to relearn how to handle normal stress and how to accept low-level anxiety and use it to my benefit. The members of this clinic have helped me accomplish these things. They have also been there with explanations for emotional and mood changes I experienced as my life moved further and further away from cigarettes. These changes did not occur all at once when I initially quit smoking. Rather, they occurred at various times throughout the entire quitting experience. I believe my ability to successfully quit is 100 percent due to the support I receive from the staff of this clinic. On my own, I never would have succeeded (I have proof of this). I would like to finish by saying that I have taken up jogging and because I don't smoke, I can now jog/run 3 miles 2 to 3 times a week (my lungs really do not hurt). Not too shabby for a non-athletic 52 year old.

Quitting. A year ago I watched helplessly as my addiction to cigarettes drained my bank account, left my room, clothes and hair and even my skin stinking of tobacco, and perhaps worst of all is the slightest physical activity became overwhelming exertion, compelling me to stop and rest in the course of journeys just down the street. I came to the smoking cessation clinic because I wanted all that to end.

I knew there was no good reason to keep smoking and that the earlier in life I could rein in my problem the easier I'd find that experience. But at first it seemed hopeless. Cigarettes were like an extension of my arm, their smoke felt as essential as oxygen. At first my attempts to quit didn't amount to more than maybe a day's unsettling struggle. I would find myself hitting the street at midnight in search of a smoke to bum. I felt like it was heroin I was addicted to, like I had a scene of withdrawal and just let the cigarettes own me, let myself wait to be ravaged by them so severely I could no longer muster the strength to strike a match. And really I must admit, after the first few attempts, I simply gave up. I wanted to avoid that feeling of overwhelming need more than I wanted to take control of my body, my mind and my finances.

I kept coming to the smoking cessation clinic, however I felt I was a hopeless case, but wasn't ready to admit it to those who seemed optimistic about my chances of success. And then, one day, it was rather like the sea just parted, and at last I could see a clear path of self control. I've thought about it long and hard, tried to identify that trigger that finally allowed me to beat back a vicious habit with nearly a 10 year grip on me. I think I concluded that the patch and the inhaler were crucial, I couldn't have done it without their substitution for those little sticks of hell, but what made the biggest difference, what allowed me to even give those tools a whole-hearted try, was the counseling. Having someone direct me on their use, encourage me to shift my dependence, analyze my hang ups, and most of all seem to have a stake in my success. Looking around the rest of life I didn't see many people telling me to just quit. My mom smokes, my roommates smoked, I was forever chatting with strangers on the street who I had little more than a shared dependency in common with. Even the friends I had who didn't smoke weren't putting any pressure on me to call it quits, likely fearing a smoker's wrath. What the practitioners provided was never pressure however. They simply gave me a pivotal excuse to finally take care of myself.

Cheryl Ragonesi: Project Coordinator and Social Worker

Tell me and I forget. Teach me and I remember. Involve me and I learn.

—Benjamin Franklin

In August 2001 I became the project coordinator of the Community Voices–Legacy Smoking Cessation project. Being a new graduate social worker, I was very green, impatient, and enthusiastic. Fortunately, I was surrounded by a team of mentors and peers who were experienced, calm, and as enthusiastic as I was. I was involved in every aspect of the project, and as the years progressed and the project unfolded I became less green and a bit more patient—but I remained as enthusiastic as on day 1. What follows is the story of my work at one of the program sites, the Mannie L. Wilson Towers in Harlem.

After visiting the site, I decided I wanted to run a support group for seniors who lived at the towers and wanted to quit smoking. "This will be easy," I thought. "I'll have the group sessions right in the community room in the same building where the seniors reside." Little did I know that that idea was the best one I had!

I made cute, colorful flyers and posted them all over the senior residence. A few weeks later, I was informed by the social worker that none of the seniors wanted to come to my group. This surprised me, so I asked why. She said, "You're scaring the seniors. You may want to change the flyers to say something like 'a support group that will help you cut down on smoking'—not to quit!" She went on to say that "Most of the residents here have been smoking longer than you have been alive, who are you to tell them they should quit?" Good point, I thought. So I changed the flyers, promised good food, and hoped for the best. Ten seniors came.

I used a cognitive behavioral model incorporating social support to test the feasibility of providing group smoking cessation sessions for seniors. Ten self-identified smokers volunteered to participate in weekly group sessions over four months. Attendance at each group session averaged 80 percent. As a result of the intervention, 10 percent of the participants quit smoking and 80 percent reported reductions in tobacco use. The lessons learned from this program include not only the importance of group settings, but also the need to know the group that you are targeting, and to tailor your expectations to meet their needs. If you incorporate these principles, the group format can be a powerful one that enhances support, promotes socialization, and helps lessen the isolation that is one of the main triggers in older smokers.

The following story of a patient's progress and struggles after many sessions at the Tobacco Cessation Clinic was written from my point of view on the clinical staff. I, along with all of the clinical staff, was humbled by the courage and grace of many of the patients. The case illustrated below is just one example of the many lives we had the privilege to be a small part of.

MR. T'S STORY

When Mr. T first presented to the clinic we were all taken aback. Picture this: a man in his mid- to late sixties, covered in buttons from head to toe. Buttons with the American flag, buttons with smiley faces, buttons with all kinds of sayings stretching from East to West in philosophical thought. I cannot tell you exactly what they said—it was prudent to keep a safe distance. Alongside Mr. T was his shopping cart filled with paper and possessions held dear.

Mr. T's medical history: Edentulous (toothless), diabetes, high cholesterol, heart condition, psychiatric comorbidity

- Mr. T's Medications: aspirin 81 mg, Gabapentin 100 mg, Mitzapine 15 mg, Xalantan (1drop each eye), Lipitor 40 mg, Glipizide 10 mg, Timolol
- Mr. T's living arrangements: When Mr. T presented to the clinic he lived in a residential facility.
- 1 pack a day smoker

When Mr. T sat down to tell us he wanted to quit smoking, quite frankly none of us believed he would be able to do it. We based our false assessment on the present circumstances, which we felt were not stacked in his favor. They were as follows: (a) He lived in a residential home where not only the residents smoked, but so did most of the counselors and group leaders. (b) His psychiatric comorbidity was so evident, and we were not sure he was on the right medications. He was incoherent at the inception of his treatment. (c) He had little social support, and those who did support him wanted him to buy them cigarettes.

Mr. T came in every week, and little by little he proved us wrong. He began to go to church and build a support system. He started using the

(Continued)

Nicotrol Inhaler, and after much instruction he began to use it correctly. He quit! Mr. T left the Tobacco Cessation Clinic a couple of months after quitting.

About one year later Mr. T presented to the clinic again. He was wearing clean pants and shirt and suit jacket. No buttons! Again, we were taken aback. Mr. T came back to us because he had relapsed. He had many changes going on, and although they were positive changes, they still caused him stress. Mr. T started the inhaler again and quit in no time at all. Mr. T now lives in a new residential facility where he has his own "smoke-free room" and his own phone and is more independent. He looks, sounds, and acts like a new man. We are so fond and proud of Mr. T. He still comes in occasionally for a booster session to report progress in his life, and pride in his continuing achievement of staying tobacco-free. By the way, we made him a referral, and he got some new teeth!

Youth Mini-Grant Programs

Don't worry that children never listen to you; worry that they are always watching you.

—Robert Fulghum

Our partnership with Alianza Dominicana, a long-standing asset to the Dominican community of New York City, ensured that the youth component of the program would reach out to a large number of the population through a trusted and well-established community organization. This organization oversaw mini-grants for the Legacy program that were distributed to community and faith-based organizations with a youth component. The youth community health worker employed by Alianza provided leadership and offered ongoing technical assistance to the youth grantees in both Washington Heights and Harlem. Other community health workers also participated in training that helped us to build organizational capacity and further the goal of empowering participating youth. As a group, the community health workers conducted a variety of activities. These included having regular meetings with each organization's youth, providing feedback on the design of the initiative, helping facilitate the process of implementation of the organizations' tobacco prevention activities or events, coordinating trainings on youth leadership, facilitating tobacco prevention workshops, and hosting an end-of-the-grant event to highlight the youths' accomplishments.

One of the most poignant experiences for the clinical staff was how personal this message was for many of the youth who participated in the minigrants. For example, one young man had a father who died from the effects of tobacco, and several others had family members who were current smokers. They often spoke about their worry and concern for their loved ones. All the youth knew someone, either a family member or a friend, who smoked. It was humbling to us to see how many young people were directly affected by tobacco in some way. It was also evident that we had a long road ahead. Although all of these services increased the credibility and visibility of the Community Voices–Legacy Smoking Cessation project, our greatest hope is that they left a mark on the youth that is indelible.

The Tobacco-Cessation Clinic at the College of Dental Medicine

> Energy and persistence conquer all things.
>
> —Benjamin Franklin

The Columbia University Tobacco Cessation Clinic takes a bio-psycho-social approach in assessing tobacco dependence and in developing individual treatment plans. This model views addiction as the complex interaction of three factors: the individual, the environment, and the drug itself. We assess the psychology (behavioral conditioning) of tobacco addiction by monitoring a sample of each smoker's environmental and emotional triggers. These are stimuli (external situational or internal subjective to the person) associated with current smoking behavior. The clinician then uses these triggers to evaluate potential future relapse back to smoking after cessation. Developing alternative behavioral strategies to smoking is a key component to preparing for a quit day and to helping promote the individual's subsequent adjustment after cessation. We also assess the social environment of the smoker by identifying others (friends, spouses, supervisors, coworkers) who smoke openly in his or her environment. It is important to note here that New York State laws that were put into place allowing for smoke-free working environments and eateries have helped many of the clients over the past four years.

Outcomes

A description of the Columbia University Tobacco Cessation Clinic and an evaluation of the program were published in 2002. We now have a more recent program evaluation from 2007 and have provided a comparison in table 6.1.

In both 2002 and 2007, one-third of the patients in the clinic were male, and two-thirds were female. In the five years from 2002 to 2007, there was a 5 percent increase in psychiatric comorbidity in the clinic patients, from 56.9 percent to 62 percent. There was no change in the percentage of patients presenting with a medical illness, which remained at 82 percent. The most striking change is in the increased success in the clinic's treatment outcomes, from 24 percent in 2002 to 68 percent in 2007. The clinic population remains a largely low socioeconomic and immigrant population, which highlights the importance of these outcomes even further. Two changes happened between the first sample of patients, seen over a six-month period in 1999, and the second sample, seen throughout 2007. First, New York State changed its Medicaid policy to cover a six-month course of smoking cessation medications. Second, the clinic's cognitive-behavioral smoking cessation therapy evolved. Based on our 2002 program evaluation, we began to train our patients to return for more help (booster sessions) before relapsing (after which they often felt ashamed and were lost to follow-up). We encouraged

TABLE 6.1

Columbia University Tobacco Cessation Clinic Demographics and Outcomes, 2002 versus 2007

	2002	2007
Gender: male	37.3%	38%
Gender: female	62.7%	62%
Mean age	52.8	49.5
Comorbid psychiatric symptoms	56.9%	62%
Medically ill	82.3%	82%
Quit at 3–12 month follow-up (only for those patients reached at follow-up)		24%
Quit at 6–12 month follow-up (for all patients seen in 2007)		68%

them to come in when they experienced an increase in cravings to smoke and thoughts about smoking. Using the community health worker model described in the next section, we improved our patient follow-up and thus improved our overall treatment outcomes.

The Role of Community Health Workers in the Tobacco Cessation Clinic

The community health workers in the tobacco cessation clinic served a different, but complementary, role from that of the youth initiative community health workers profiled earlier in this chapter. Initial plans for the clinic did not include a community health worker but relied instead on a translator. It was recognized early on that the translator had in fact taken on a more comprehensive CHW role. Subsequently, the role of translator and community health worker became a single enlarged role and proved to be an essential component in the successful implementation of the Community Voices–Legacy program. The activities carried out by the clinic CHW included extensive community outreach, intake and assessment, referrals and case management, social support, informal counseling, provision of specialized education, and follow-up care. The role of the CHW in the Community Voices–Legacy program became critical to reach out to underserved populations who were interested in receiving counseling. More so, CHW was extremely important in maintaining ongoing relationships with patients and providing follow-up care after the initial contact with the clinic staff.

As documented by the clinic community health workers, the following strategies were employed to encourage participation at the Tobacco Cessation Clinic:

1. Emphasize that language would not be a barrier since a bilingual translator was available.
2. To ensure attendance at follow-up appointments, contact patients over the phone the day before their appointment.
3. Give referrals as needed to other social services, and make information available about other clinics and community agencies when necessary.
4. Contact the clients' pharmacist when they confronted problems in filling their smoking cessation prescriptions, a not infrequent occurrence.

In addition, it was important to maintain active communication with community partners. For example, culturally appropriate information about the services available was sent out on a consistent basis.

Martin Ovalles, Tobacco Cessation Clinic CHW

I could not have imagined a better way to learn about the health care system in general, and tobacco cessation in particular, than the opportunity given to me at the Tobacco Cessation Clinic at Columbia University Medical Center.

During my last semester in college (fall 1999) majoring in psychology, I had the option to do an internship. I contacted Lynn Tepper at the Behavioral Medicine Program at Columbia University College of Dental Medicine and asked her to give me the opportunity to volunteer at the Tobacco Cessation Clinic for the semester. She introduced me to the director, Daniel Seidman, and told him about my interest in helping out with anything I could. They decided I could help as a translator, a role that evolved over time into my present role as clinic community health worker.

After completing my internship, I was so impressed with what I had learned from such a terrific team that I asked Dr. Seidman if I could continue volunteering at the clinic. His approval was as gratifying as if I had landed a well-paid job. The staff from the clinic may have thought I was doing them a favor, but I was the one who benefited from the vast experience of each of them.

After two years, I was presented with the opportunity to be part of the Legacy Foundation grant for the next four years. This enabled me to be part of an extraordinary journey during which the clinic ascended to the next level. Our participation in health fairs throughout the city was a huge success. It was an excellent channel to provide people with more information about us and how to get to the clinic. The time to see patients was extended, and reliability with follow-up appointments improved remarkably. Patients seemed to enjoy the fact that every time they came to visit us we always had the same team waiting for them. Indeed, one of the reasons Spanish-speaking patients do not like to come back for follow-up visits is that they often have to share their personal stories with a different translator and/or clinician. When the Legacy grant ended, I was fortunate enough to be hired by the Columbia University College of Dental Medicine to remain a part of the Tobacco Cessation Clinic.

Nowadays I am still doing my best to help people quit smoking. I am working as a behavioral interventionist on a National Institutes of Health grant at the Naomi Berrie Diabetes Center. Thanks to the Tobacco Cessation Clinic, I have developed the set of skills I need to teach adolescents how to better manage behavioral aspects of their diabetes. It has not always been easy, but I will never be able to quantify the many benefits I have received since the very first day I came to the clinic asking for an opportunity to do my college internship.

Daniel Seidman, M.D.: Lessons Learned and Discussion

As the director of the Columbia University Medical Center Tobacco Cessation Clinic, I have been privileged to watch our staff and trainees grow and change as we learn and evolve as a clinical service and training program. Our growth as clinicians mirrors the growth and changes we see in our patients as we learn from them how best to help them overcome their smoking addiction. Our evolving but stable relationship to our patients and the community we are serving also helps us to follow up with our patients as they make healthy life changes to prevent relapse.

Historically, dependence on cigarettes and tobacco has not been viewed as a clinical disorder requiring professional assistance. To cite one example, the American Cancer Society served for many years as the major community resource to help smokers in the New York City area. Under the circumstances their Fresh Start program did a great job. The American Cancer Society employed volunteers who were ex-smokers but who had no professional training as group leaders. In addition, no assessments of participants were done, and no medical or psychological expertise was offered. The American Cancer Society ended the program in New York City in 1998.

The kind of lay approach exemplified by Fresh Start can no longer suffice as the mainstay in helping smokers quit. For a variety of reasons, it has now become increasingly crucial that the health professions actively take up treatment of their tobacco-dependent patients as a key part of their mission. First, over the last two decades or so perceptions of smoking as recreational, or just a bad habit, have changed, with increasing public awareness of tobacco dependence as a serious addictive disorder. Second, new developments such as nicotine replacement therapies, Zyban, and more effective psychological counseling and behavioral strategies such as cognitive-behavioral therapy have dramatically changed what is available to help smokers quit. Third, it has become increasingly clear that many people still addicted to smoking have comorbid psychiatric conditions such as depression, alcoholism, or schizophrenia. An astounding 41 percent of people who reported having mental illness in the past month were current smokers and represented 40.6 percent of all current smokers in the United States (Lasser et al. 2000). This study estimated that people with mental illness comprised 44.3 percent of the U.S. tobacco market. And finally, there are now quite excellent standards for smoking cessation treatment available, which are based on careful review of the vast empirical literature (Fiore 2000; Fiore et al. 1996; Fiore et al. 2008). These guidelines are ripe to become a baseline against which the health professions will be held accountable in the future. For these and many other reasons, health care professionals can no longer rightly leave the care of tobacco addiction to well-meaning nonprofessionals from the community. The success of the Northern Manhattan Community Voices Collaborative has been precisely the integration of the community health worker into the university-based Tobacco Cessation Clinic. This effort effectively brings the best available clinical approaches to the community; it does not wait for the community to come to us in the medical center but offers a consistent team approach to encourage community members' participation in the clinical work by making this as comfortable for them as possible.

The lives that have been affected by this program are countless. In this chapter, we could give only a sampling. From the project staff, to the youth leaders, to the clients we served at the clinic, the program has had a life-changing effect that will continue to benefit the northern Manhattan community.

Editors' note: The NMCVC did most of its work in beginning new initiatives in the 1998 to 2003–2005 period. The idea was to build capacity in partner institutions and/or create new leadership to keep the initiatives going. The tobacco initiative described in this chapter was designed in part to spread the Tobacco Cessation Clinic first begun in the College of Dental Medicine into the off-site centers of New York Presbyterian Hospital; hence, the effort to educate the leadership of the off-site clinics. However, we just learned that in 2009 New York State changed its Medicaid policy on reimbursement for tobacco counseling. Seidman provides his perspective on this change in policy:

We have demonstrated that innovative tobacco cessation services can help low-income smokers who have multiple medical, psychiatric, and dental problems. These patients are unlikely to respond to brief interventions offered in the primary care setting: in fact, most of the patients we worked with in our clinics had already been through one or more unsuccessful regimens of smoking cessation medications with physician or dentist counseling. Yet they were nonetheless motivated to come to the tobacco cessation clinic. Many of these smokers are high users of medical and dental services, and their continued smoking places an enormous economic burden on the health care system, undermining the ongoing efforts of so many health professionals.

Over the years of running the Tobacco Cessation Clinic, we forged a general agreement among the medical, psychiatric, and dental leadership at our medical center that these specialized tobacco cessation services are a valuable part of what is required by a rational health care delivery system. Yet, despite this widespread recognition, funding models for the health care system do not provide ongoing resources for the kind of comprehensive cognitive-behavioral treatment described in this chapter, and which we believe is required by a significant subpopulation of smokers. In the current health care environment, where every dollar must be accounted for, no institution can afford to run any program—no matter how valuable or essential—if it is not financially self-sustaining.

In light of the current budget realities at the end of 2008, the Tobacco Cessation Clinic we described in this chapter was closed. Although New York State Medicaid pays for smoking cessation medications (covering two three-month trials in a twelve-month period), as of 2009 Medicaid explicitly denies coverage for counseling to go along with these medications, with the one exception of pregnant women. Sadly, despite support from the Obama administration for $75 million in funding for smoking cessation on the national level, some politicians and journalists labeled spending on smoking cessation as "frivolous" and "wasteful" according to the *New York Times* (February 2, 2009). And despite a growing recognition among those on the frontlines of delivering health care of the critical need to address smokers with multiple morbidities (e.g., serious psychiatric, medical, and dental illnesses), the reality is that the public funding and political support for this approach are just not there at the present time.

So, the achievements described in this chapter remain to be realized as part of a future transformation of the health care delivery system where comprehensive clinical treatment, and prevention, of smoking addiction are truly recognized and supported as a valued service.

References

Alianza Dominicana (1995). *Focus group final report.*

Fiore, M. (2000). A clinical practice guideline for treating tobacco use and dependence. A U.S. Public Health Service Report. *JAMA* 283, no. 24: 3244–54.

Fiore, M., et al. (1996). *Smoking cessation: Clinical practice guideline no. 18.* AHCPR publication 96–0692. Rockville, Md.: U.S. Department of Health and Human Services, Public Health Service, Agency for Health Care Policy and Research.

Fiore, M.C., et al. (2008). *Treating tobacco use and dependence: 2008 update. Clinical practice guideline.* Rockville, Md.: U.S. Department of Health and Human Services, Public Health Service.

Lasser, K., et al. (2000). Smoking and mental illness: a population-based prevalence study. *JAMA* 284, no. 20: 2606–10.

Seidman, D. F., et al. (2002). Serving underserved and hard-core smokers in a dental school setting. *Journal of Dental Education* 66, no. 4: 507–13.

U.S. Department of Health and Human Services. (1999). *National survey results on drug use from the Monitoring the Future Study, 1975–1998,* vol. 1: *Secondary school students.* NIH Pub. no. 99-4660. Washington, D.C.: National Institute on Drug Abuse.

Selected Additional References

Borrell-Carrió, F., A. L. Suchman, and R. M. Epstein (2004). The biopsychosocial model 25 years later: Principles, practice, and scientific inquiry. *Annals of Family Medicine* 2, no. 6: 576–82.

New York City Housing Development Corporation (2009). "HDC and the West Harlem Group Assistance Celebrate the Re-opening of the Mannie L. Wilson Towers Senior Residence." http://newyork.realestaterama.com/2009/06/25/hdc-and-the-west-harlem-group-assistance-celebrate-the-reopening-of-the-mannie-l-wilson-towers-senior-residence-ID0720.html.

New York State Department of Health (n.d.). "Information for a Healthy New York: Tobacco Cessation Centers." http://www.health.state.ny.us/prevention/tobacco_control/community_partners/tobacco_cessation_centers.htm.

Smoke Free Society (2007) "Peter Jennings dies of lung cancer." http://www.smokefreesociety.org/NewsClip/Jennings-3.asp.

Part III

Strengthening the Safety Net

This part presents NMCVC projects for systems changes to provide a primary care home for patients seeking routine care in the emergency room; improve the capacity of community-based organizations to easily find health care facilities for uninsured clients via an interactive website; and use the public school system to educate parents and children about healthy food and exercise choices. Efforts to develop a new insurance product for the uninsured in northern Manhattan are also covered.

[7]

Salud a Su Alcance (SASA)

Health Within Your Reach

ANITA LEE

The health care access problem is not the lack of programs. Rather, it is the lack of responsiveness of these programs to the needs of the very people they were funded to serve.

Salud a Su Alcance (SASA), which is Spanish for "Health Care Within Your Reach," was created with funding from the Health Resources and Services Administration under its Healthy Community Access Program Initiative during 2001–2004. The purpose of the initiative was to seed the development of sustainable solutions that address the health disparities among uninsured populations. One grant requirement was the formation of a coalition that would contribute resources and diverse expertise to ensure the sustainability of program activities. SASA was formed to satisfy that requirement.

The original partners of the SASA Coalition included New York Presbyterian Hospital, which was the lead organization; the Northern Manhattan Community Voices Collaborative of Columbia University; and Alianza Dominicana. As the program evolved, the SASA Coalition expanded to include three federally qualified health centers: Morris Heights Health Center, Community Healthcare Network, and Urban Health Plan.

SASA's overarching vision consisted of three components. The first was to foster a strong partnership among diverse key stakeholders to bridge the service gaps for the uninsured population. The second was to "fix" the fragmented health care system. The third was to create a sustainable infrastructure that would continue the research for innovative strategies for a seamless neighborhood health and social system that is responsive to the needs of residents.

Our three original strategies were:

1. Increase enrollment into public insurance.
2. Connect people to a medical home and other referral services.
3. Divert people from the emergency department to more appropriate care settings.

These strategies were selected based on the assumption that people without insurance do not have a medical home and will use the emergency department as their primary source of care. Therefore our top priority was to enroll eligible people into Medicaid and find them a medical home, hence eliminating the need for using the emergency department for non-acute episodes (table 7.1).

TABLE 7.1

Making a Difference: SASA

PROBLEMS

Uninsured lack access to health services
Inappropriate use of emergency department for primary care
Pharmaceutical gap for uninsured patients
People with diabetes overuse emergency department

SOLUTIONS

Key partner Alianza Dominicana trained five facilitated enrollment specialists
  Provider referral hotline
CARE, a three-pronged strategy to identify "frequent flyer" patients, provide
  targeted intervention, and offer care management
SAS–PAP helped access donated drugs
SAS–DMP trained 5 CHWs to work with patients

RESULTS

30,000 uninsured people enrolled in public health programs
Bilingual staff person provided links to health care and cut through red tape
95% reduction in emergency department utilization
2,000 patients obtained 10,000 prescriptions (worth $5 million)
Significant reductions in A1c and LDL levels

What We Did and How and Why We Did It

In 2001 I became the program director of SASA. Although I have a background in community health program design, I had little preconceived notion of Washington Heights/Inwood as a community or the characteristics of Dominicans, who make up the majority of the population in that section of northern Manhattan. My lack of knowledge about the community and the target population made me operate with a humble and open mind. The experience that I had acquired as a former public health advisor for the U.S. Public Health Service taught me to approach problems with simple, pragmatic solutions. Washington Heights/Inwood, like most ethnic enclaves in New York, is composed of low-income minorities where most adults are monolingual with low-paying jobs. While struggling daily with life stressors, the residents attempt to navigate a very complicated health care and social system for themselves and their families. To ensure that our strategy is effective, we followed three guiding principles when developing our programs:

1. *Build trust.* We deployed local human resources who were eager to learn and help. The staff of SASA, for the most part, represented the communities we served. They were the trusted liaisons between the community and the health care system, informants for the health care system, health educators, and patient advocates.

2. *Perpetuate reconnaissance.* Before we crafted a solution, we first sought to understand why the problem existed and what strategies would have a greater chance of success. Instead of conducting focus groups, organizing fact-finding forums, or surveying our community, we asked each staff member to listen, explore, and probe when engaging the patients. This has proven to be the most important and valuable approach and has given us many "ah-ha" and "duh" moments.

3. *Keep solutions simple and quick.* We made a deliberate effort to respond to each patient's needs expeditiously with simple solutions that required minimal hand-offs (patient being passed from one person to the next). We evaluated short-term results immediately. Strategies that demonstrated positive results were memorialized as procedures and communicated to key stakeholders in the health care system to be adopted and institutionalized.

Each partner of the SASA Coalition represented a different sector of the health care system. New York Presbyterian Hospital is the leading academic medical center, one of the largest health care systems in New York City, and the largest employer of the community. The Mailman School of Public Health, a higher education institution that supported research and evaluation of public and community health projects, was also a partner in the Kellogg Community Voices grant. Alianza Dominicana is a multiservice social service agency that is rooted in the Washington Heights community. These were eventually joined by three federally qualified health centers whose mission is to provide comprehensive preventive and primary care services regardless of patients' ability to pay.

In the first year of implementation, SASA embarked on the Insurance Enrollment, Provider Referral Hotline, and Emergency Department Diversion projects. These three projects seemed to be the most direct and logical solutions in addressing the lack of access to health services for people with no health insurance. The lessons learned in the first year led to the development and implementation of the Pharmacy Assistance and Diabetes Management programs.

Insurance Enrollment Program

Alianza Dominicana was the key partner in the Insurance Enrollment program. It provided five facilitated enrollment specialists who were stationed in strategic locations in New York Presbyterian Hospital's community-based practices and emergency room to assess every uninsured person's eligibility for Medicaid or other public insurance. Unexpectedly, the 2001 attack on the World Trade Center led to the authorization of the Disaster Relief Medicaid program, allowing any New York City resident to qualify for one year of Medicaid. Between 2001 and 2003 Alianza Dominicana enrolled thirty thousand people in health insurance programs. This gave us a jump-start that helped us capture a fairly substantial group of people who later became ineligible for Medicaid. (See chapter 3 for more about facilitated enrollment successes.)

Provider Referral Hotline

The Provider Referral Hotline was set up for patients, advocates, and community physicians seeking a medical home, specialty care, or diagnostic services. One bilingual staff person established linkages with hospital outpatient clinics, federally qualified health centers, and community physicians to facilitate appointment scheduling and advise patients in preparing the required documentation to qualify for a sliding fee scale and getting past all the health care system red tape.

Care Coordination, Advocacy, Reconnaissance, and Education (CARE)

CARE is our emergency department diversion project, and is also the cornerstone of the SASA Coalition. This three-pronged strategy employed a technology to identify "frequent flyer" patients, provided targeted intervention, and offered care management. The process began with a proprietary software called *Vigilens*, which is an event-monitoring technology developed in collaboration with the Columbia University Department of Medical Informatics. *Vigilens* tagged any patient in the hospital's data warehouse who had visited the emergency department three or more times in the past six months for ambulatory care sensitive diagnosis. When the patient visited the emergency department again, an email alert was sent to a health priority specialist who contacted the patient within twenty-four hours to begin a series of telephone assessments and consultations. The initial phone conversation included an assessment of circumstances that led to the frequent emergency department visits. Once the immediate barriers were identified, the health priority specialist responded with a direct and expeditious intervention to eliminate those barriers, such as getting the patient public insurance, facilitating an appointment with a primary care provider or a specialist, helping the patient understand how to use the Medicaid managed care plan, or simply letting patients know that the emergency department is not where one should seek primary care. Other barriers and life stressors, such as self-management of diabetes and other chronic conditions, elimination of asthma triggers in the home, and identification of psychosocial and legal problems and appropriate referrals to mental health and social service agencies, were addressed in the subsequent phone calls. CARE generated some astounding results. Available data show that 620 "frequent flyers" identified by *Vigilens* generated a total of 2,784 emergency department visits (4.5 visits/person) over six months prior to our intervention. These patients received an initial call from the health priority specialist, then two more calls at three-month intervals to reinforce messages and address new barriers. At the end of nine months, the emergency department utilization rate was reduced to 0.38 visits per person. This represented a *95 percent reduction in emergency department utilization* over a nine-month period!

The success of this program was attributed to the two health priority specialists, both foreign medical graduates from the Dominican Republic, who applied the three guiding principles of SASA in their assessments and interventions: listening to the patients, promptly mobilizing the resources from the hospital and partnering agencies to address every barrier presented to them, and diligently following up to ensure that the barriers have been dealt with. CARE became the information vault. Even though the information was anecdotal, it helped weave a tapestry of stories with faces and pulses that blanketed the bodegas, the tenements, and the limousines of Washington Heights and Inwood. There are similar stories that can surface in every ethnic enclave in New York City, varied only in color and language.

SASA–Pharmacy Assistance Program (SASA–PAP)

When Disaster Relief Medicaid expired in 2002, many patients lost their Medicaid due to lack of legal resident status or income exceeding the Medicaid income limits. Many of these patients had been diagnosed with chronic conditions and had just started their treatment regimen. Along with their temporary Medicaid coverage, the prescription coverage that enabled them to continue therapeutic treatment for their chronic conditions was abruptly terminated. Although most primary care providers in the SASA network continued to provide low-cost medical care to these uninsured patients, none offered any assistance for pharmaceuticals. SASA responded to the pharmaceutical gap by creating the SASA–Pharmacy Assistance Program (SASA–PAP). SASA–PAP was the first program in New York City that helped safety net providers access donated drugs for eligible uninsured patients. With two full-time staff, this program helped more than two thousand patients obtain over ten thousand prescriptions from over 180 major pharmaceutical manufacturers' Indigent Drug programs—for a total worth of $5 million. This program continues to operate in New York Presbyterian Hospital, serving more than three hundred safety net providers. In an effort to expand the capacity and reach of SASA–PAP, I cultivated a partnership with the New York City Department of Health and Mental Hygiene to develop NYCRx, a nonprofit organization governed by safety net providers. The mission was to make available affordable drugs for low-income New Yorkers by expanding the use of the 340B federal drug discount program and access to other low-cost pharmaceuticals.

SASA–Diabetes Management Program (SASA–DMP)

Despite the interventions by our health priority specialists, we found that one group of frequent flyers continued to return to the emergency department: those diagnosed with diabetes. SASA, in its third and final year of funding, responded with the SASA–Diabetes Management Program (SASA–DMP). A1C level is a measure of how well diabetes is controlled, so we asked our network providers to refer any patient with an A1C level of 10 or higher to SASA–DMP for case management. We trained and recruited five community health workers to conduct home visits to teach patients self-management techniques, coordinate their care, coach patients and families in adopting healthy lifestyles, and connect the patients to health and social services.

Patients who enrolled in SASA–DMP were assigned a community health worker to assess their living conditions, knowledge of diabetes, and understanding of how to manage their diabetes and other comorbidities. The community health workers, all recruited from local community-based organizations and trained by New York Presbyterian Hospital's staff, were resources for community and health system services. Community health workers helped patients set personal self-management goals, one goal at a time, and worked with the patients and family members for up to six months. At the end of six months, 80 percent of the enrollees demonstrated an average of 8 percent reduction in A1C, and 31 percent demonstrated an 8 percent reduction of low-density lipoprotein cholesterol (LDL, considered to be the "bad" cholesterol); after three months of intervention, 44 percent of the enrollees demonstrated a 15 percent reduction in LDL. (Chapter 3 tells the bigger story of the community health workers.)

What Did We Accomplish?

If we measured SASA's success based on the programs' sustainability, then it was immensely successful. The insurance enrollment project was sustained by Medicaid Managed Care Organizations. These organizations have invested substantial amount of funds in outreach and marketing efforts, enrolling eligible uninsured people on street corners and in clinics. On any given day, one could stumble on at least five enrollment vans from various Medicaid Managed Care Organizations saturating low-income neighborhoods.

The one-staff referral center that connected patients to medical homes and diagnostic and specialty services has been expanded to a call center with six operators expediting primary, specialty, and diagnostic appointments for patients. Uninsured patients can now obtain a primary care appointment at New York Presbyterian Hospital's Ambulatory Care Network at a discount through this call center.

CARE remains the most talked-about SASA project. This much-acclaimed program eliminated a common myth that uninsured patients represent the majority of frequent flyers who use the emergency room for nonacute episodes. Over a three-year period CARE demonstrated that only 6 percent of the frequent flyers identified were uninsured: more than 68 percent were Medicaid managed-care and Medicaid patients. The success of CARE in diverting emergency department visits would result in the reduction of billable Medicaid visits. As a result, CARE was financially unappealing to the hospital and the Medicaid Managed Care organizations. Unfortunately, CARE was not sustainable because of inherent flaws within the reimbursement system established by both government and private payers. The system does not offer any incentive for providers to contain cost and coordinate care for its members; instead, it provides the opportunity to perpetuate abuse. But there is always a silver lining around every dark cloud. In 2004 Dr. Walid Michelen, the principal investigator of SASA, transferred the CARE strategy to Lincoln Hospital, which holds a full-risk managed care contract with its primary Medicaid HMO, Metro Plus. The CARE project, which has taken a life of its own under Dr. Michelen's direction, has consistently generated an average annual savings of $350,000 in avoided emergency room care. In addition, the project was expanded to prevent inappropriate admissions. This has resulted in savings of an average of $800,000 a year in unnecessary admissions.

Because SASA–DMP's evaluation demonstrated improvements of clinical outcome measures among its participants, it has been used to support and validate the effectiveness of community health workers in chronic disease management. The results of this program have stimulated interest among community health worker advocacy groups, managed care organizations, community-based organizations, health centers, hospital ambulatory care providers, and even pharmaceutical companies. SASA was one of the pioneers in deploying local resources and building community capacity by developing community health workers to support disease management programs and integrate the community and cultural elements with clinical best practices to improve patient health outcomes. Health care providers, helpless as they are watching the rise in the prevalence of diabetes and the incidence of diabetes-related death, have been inspired by SASA–DMP. Managed care organizations and health care institutions are collaborating with community-based organizations to replicate the SASA–DMP strategy in battling diabetes. The community health worker diabetes training program and tools have seeded many community health worker programs in northern Manhattan. Borrowing the findings and proven strategies used by SASA–DMP, Alianza Dominicana and Northern Manhattan Perinatal Partnership, two major community-based organizations serving northern Manhattan, were separately awarded grants to replicate various components of SASA–DMP.

Despite these positive outcomes, SASA did not change the health care system. After three years, SASA found several strategies that filled some service gaps, eradicated some myths, and uncovered many flaws within the health care system. Our solutions, however, were merely Band-Aids for a health care system that is hemorrhaging as a result of uncontrollable cost, special interests, and inherent inefficiency.

HEALTH CARE STORIES

While writing this chapter, many dialogues and faces resurfaced, each telling their own story. These stories reflect the good, the bad, and the ugly of the health care system. In spite of our mixed experiences, the SASA staff and I felt privileged that we were part of these stories.

(Continued)

Story 1: I was riding in a limousine going to New York Presbyterian Hospital. The driver showed me his swollen ankle and asked if I could find him a doctor. When I asked him if he had applied for Medicaid or Family Health Plus, he showed me his Family Health Plus card and stated that he did not know what to do with it. I took a close look at his insurance card and found the name of his primary care physician and her telephone number on the back of the card in 8-font print. I called that number for him from my cell phone, but no one answered the phone. There was not even an opportunity to leave a message. The driver never received any information on how to use this life-saving card that was simply sent to him by mail. Crucial information was obscured in small print. I was left wondering whether this was a result of poor service or a deliberate effort to deny access.

Story 2: The Pharmacy Assistance program assisted a 55-year-old Dominican man who was getting medical care at the one of New York Presbyterian's ambulatory care clinics to obtain seven medications for his hypertension, ulcers, arthritis, depression, and asthma. Two months later, the patient was given a referral slip by the hospital social worker to transfer his care to the nearest public hospital because he was "uninsurable." Given that our "secure network" did not include the city hospital, we would not be able to continue to provide pharmaceutical assistance for him if he obtained medical care outside of the network. We tried to refer the patient to our two FQHC partners, but care was denied due to "lack of documentation to place him on a sliding fee scale." Our resourceful health priority specialist finally identified a community physician who offered free medical care to this patient. For about a year, the patient received primary care from a community physician, received all his medications from SASA–PAP, and became gainfully employed as a storekeeper in a local pharmacy until he was diagnosed with cancer. This gentleman has since passed on. He had made our job meaningful.

Story 3: An elderly woman with uncontrollable diabetes living alone in West Harlem was referred to the SASA–DMP by her primary care physician at the hospital clinic. She was not compliant with her medication regime because of her inability to pay for her diabetic prescriptions. She would take selective medications only when she felt ill. After enrolling in SASA–DMP, all her medications were obtained through SASA–PAP at no cost. Her A1C level was reduced from 11 to 5.7 in six months. The SASA–DMP community health worker also helped her apply for Medicaid and home health assistance.

Lessons Learned

Several enabling factors helped us achieved our positive results. First, the demographics of the staff reflected those of our target population. Most of the SASA staff and community health workers lived in Washington Heights and the South Bronx. They contributed their personal experience and knowledge to help us frame our patient communication to achieve better outcomes. Second, because SASA was a "demonstration project" and not a research project with strictly defined protocols, we tweaked our program continuously during its operation to adjust our strategies and approaches. Third, although the SASA programs were designed in a silo, they were implemented with cooperation and support from providers and hospital administrators.

Our most important strategy has been religiously adhering to the three guiding principles: build trust, perpetual reconnaissance, and keep the solutions simple. On a continual basis, we applied the lessons we learned from interacting with the system or the patients to improve our odds, facilitated services to our patients, pressed for actions, and continued to listen, learn, and make adjustments to our approach. We eliminated many insurmountable barriers simply by being resourceful and creative. Using a little bit of wit and having a sense of obligation also helped.

I have gained some insights about our health care system that are based primarily on my experience working on SASA during the three-year period and observations that I made over the span of my career. These insights could be summarized into three points:

1. *Health disparity is suffering from being overdiagnosed.* Health disparity is a product of our health care system. Both public and private think tanks, as well as our institutional and community leaders, have spent billions of dollars and much of their professional lives to research, debate, and create new initiatives in an attempt to eliminate health disparity. The fact is, we would have gotten much farther had we hired the single mother living in the Polo Ground Projects or the homeless man hauling emptied soda bottles on the streets of Harlem as consultants to fix our health disparity problem. We have not listened to the voices of the community—the people's voices. Their voices have been drowned out by the voices of experts and intellects eager to help them.

2. *Less is more.* A common belief resonating among experts is that the solutions to all ills of the health care system are more resources,

more programs, and more grants to fund more centers and institutes. In my recollection, the number of programs and funding continued to increase year after year. There are many more social service agencies, community health centers, and both public and private investments in the health care system now compared to ten years ago. However, the health disparity problem has, over time, become bigger and meaner. Therefore, I conclude that the fragmentation of the health care system is in large part a result of too many programs. The multitude of programs offered by health care institutions, social service organizations, government agencies, and managed care organizations are unconnected dots, at times unrelated, at times competing with one another, jammed among each other in densely populated, low-income neighborhoods. Even the most sophisticated health care professional would be humiliated and lost if asked to navigate this health care maze. The solution commonly recommended to defragment our health care system is to create a program to connect the programs. Only recently have evaluators begun to examine the return on investment of these programs. If we had fewer resources, perhaps our "partnerships," "networks," and "collaboratives" would function more efficiently. If someone begins to ask for accountability, maybe programs would be more effective and our system would achieve the sought-after integration and coordination.

3. *Could somebody just answer the phone?* I often heard our SASA staff yelling: "Forget cultural sensitivity or linguistic competence, just answer the #@%* phone and connect me to someone who cares." Because SASA staff get to walk in our patients' shoes, the most valuable lesson they learn is to experience the apathy and incompetence that our patients experience when dealing with social services agencies, community health centers, and hospitals that boast "patient-centered care." This harks back to lesson number 2: the health care access problem is not the lack of programs. Rather, it is the lack of responsiveness of these programs to the needs of the very people they were funded to serve. Irrespective of socioeconomic class, race, or culture, everyone deserves to receive timely, responsive, quality services. Government bureaucracy and inadequate resources are often blamed for the inefficiency ingrained in our health care system. When inefficiency and unresponsiveness are ignored, they become a part of the system and accepted standard of practice.

Here is just one example of how this can play out in real life. One former Medicaid patient with low English proficiency shared with me that
after she received health insurance from her employer, she transferred her
care from her community health clinic to a private practice seven miles
from her community on the posh Upper East Side, where the only person
who could communicate in her language was the medical assistant. She
felt that she was finally receiving quality care and services and no longer
had to wait three hours to see the provider. Her provider and his staff
treated her with more respect and compassion than those at the community health clinic that she called her medical home for years.

Health care researchers believe that new management concepts, operational re-engineering, technology, innovative community-based initiatives,
and evidence-based clinical practices are cures to our problem. As our
institutional executives are studying high-impact solutions such as Sigma,
Open Access, PDSA Cycles, and Balance Scorecards, terms such as health
disparity, integrated health delivery system, patient-center care, and coordinated care have been echoing everywhere for at least a decade. Uninsured patients, crowded in the perimeter, are still agonizing over how to
gain entry into our system. The community's voices we captured during
the development of SASA eventually turned into sighs of despair, cries of
anguish, whimpers of painful moans, and finally bewildered and perplexed
silence.

Developing SASA undoubtedly was one of the highlights of my career.
I have had the opportunity to work with some of the most energetic and
truly compassionate individuals I have ever met. It has been quite reward-
ing to watch the young men and women who were part of this journey
blossom into effective public health professionals. They fully immersed
themselves in the mission and contributed their talents and stamina to the
project. Most of the SASA staff have advanced to positions where they have
used the skills and experience they acquired to broaden their influence
in their respective positions. The SASA–DMP project coordinator is now a
medical quality improvement consultant for the New York City Department of Health and Mental Hygiene assisting providers in using patient
registries and electronic medical records to facilitate chronic disease management. The first SASA–PAP program coordinator is now the associate
director of strategic planning at Lincoln Hospital; the second PAP program coordinator is attending medical school in Cuba. One of the health
priority specialists is working for Lincoln Hospital replicating the CARE

Project; the other is the manager of New York Presbyterian Hospital's call center, performing triage to facilitate appointments for patients.

In closing, I want to acknowledge the hundreds of patients who have given us their trust and opportunities to provide perhaps temporarily relief of their pain and suffering or a long-lasting impact on their health. They all helped us gain a better understanding of their challenges, taught us how we can meet their needs, and patiently waited for us to learn how to do it right.

References

Andrews, J. O., et al. (2004). Use of community health workers in research with ethnic minority women. *Journal of Nursing Scholarship* 36, no. 4: 358–66.

Beckham, S., et al. (2004). A community-based asthma management program: Effects on resource utilization and quality of life. *Hawaii Medical Journal* 63, no. 4: 121–26.

Bloom, J. R., et al. (1987). Improving hypertension control through tailoring: A pilot study using selective assignment of patients to treatment approaches. *Patient Education and Counseling* 10, no. 1: 39–51.

Butz, A. M., et al. (1994). Use of community health workers with inner-city children who have asthma. *Clinical Pediatrics* 33, no. 3: 135–41.

Fedder, D. O., et al. (2003). The effectiveness of community health worker outreach program on healthcare utilization of west Baltimore City Medicaid patients with diabetes, with or without hypertension. *Ethnicity and Disease* 13, no. 1: 22–27.

Gary, T. L., et al. (2004). A randomized controlled trial of the effects of nurse case manager and community health worker team interventions in urban African-Americans with type 2 diabetes. *Control Clinical Trials* 25, no. 1: 53–66.

Goldwag, R., et al. (2002). Predictors of patient dissatisfaction with emergency care. *Israel Medical Association Journal* 4, no. 8: 603–6.

Hill, M. N., et al. (1999). A clinical trial to improve high blood pressure care in young urban black men: Recruitment, follow-up, and outcomes. *American Journal of Hypertension* 12, no. 6: 548–54.

Hripcsak, G., J. J. Cimino, and S. Sengupta (1999). Web CIS: Large-scale deployment of web-based clinical information system. *Proceedings of AMIA Symposium*: 804–8.

Love, M. B., et al. (2004). CHWs get credit: A 10-year history of the first college-credit certificate for community health workers in the United States. *Health Promotion Practice* 5, no. 4: 418–28.

Michelen, W., J. Martinez, A. Lee, and D. P. Wheeler (2006). Reducing frequent flyer emergency department visits. *Journal of Health Care for the Poor and Underserved* 17, no. 1 (Suppl.): 59–69.

Nemcek, M. A., and R. Sabatier (2003). State of evaluation: Community health workers. *Public Health Nursing* 20, no. 4: 260–70.

New York City Department of Health and Mental Hygiene (2003). *Central Harlem and Washington Heights/Inwood community health profiles*. New York: NYC DHMH.

—— (2006). *Community health profiles*. http://www.nyc.gov/html/doh/html/data/data.shtml.

New York City Mayor's Office (2004). *Public health insurance participation in the community districts of New York City*. New York City: Mayor's Office of Health Insurance Access.

Swider, S. M. (2002). Outcome effectiveness of community health workers: An integrative literature review. *Public Health Nursing* 19, no. 1: 11–20.

United Hospital Fund (2003). *New York community health atlas*. New York: United Hospital Fund.

U.S. Census Bureau (2000). *2000 census of population and housing. Summary population and housing characteristics, New York*. Pub. no. PHC-1-34. Washington, D.C.: U.S. Census Bureau.

Walker, D. G., and S. Jan (2005). How do we determine whether community health workers are cost-effective? Some core methodological issues. *Journal of Community Health* 30, no. 3: 221–29.

Zuvekas A., et al. (1999). Impact of community health workers on access, use of services, and patient knowledge and behavior. Journal of Ambulatory Care Management 22, no. 4: 33–44.

Selected Additional References

LeCouteur, E. (2004). *New York's Disaster Relief Medicaid: What Happened When It Ended?* Commonwealth Fund.

New York City Housing Authority website. http://www.nyc.gov/html/nycha/html/home/home.shtml (for information about housing projects).

NYCRx website. http://www.nycrx.org/.

New York State Department of Health. (2001). *DOH Medicaid update*, 16, no. 11.

Vigilens website at Columbia University. http://www.dbmi.columbia.edu/lussier/Vigilens.html.

[8]

Health Information Tool
for Empowerment (HITE)

Making Health Care Resources a Mouse Click Away

YISEL ALONZO

Health and social service professionals face enormous daily time pres-
sures. HITE's goal is to enhance their ability to meet the complicated
needs of their uninsured clients, and ultimately increase the health
and well-being of uninsured and underinsured New Yorkers.

—Rima Cohen, founder of HITE

In northern Manhattan, high poverty and unemployment rates, overcrowded
housing and schools, low educational achievement, language barriers, cultural misconceptions, immigration issues, and distrust of "the system"
have combined to create poor and deteriorating health conditions. Contributing to and compounding the problem is the high rate of uninsured people in most northern Manhattan neighborhoods. Despite an extensive array
of public-funded health insurance programs, in 2006 the uninsured rates
were 27 percent in East Harlem and 20 percent in Washington Heights/
Inwood, as compared to 13 percent in Manhattan overall.

Although there exist many health care providers for people who cannot
afford to pay for health care or insurance and who have special needs, the
network of health care resources available to the uninsured population is
highly fragmented, and some types of health care providers are extremely
scarce. As a result, northern Manhattan has been designated a Medical
and Dental Health Manpower Shortage Area by the Health Resources Services Administration of the Department of Health and Human Services.
The tragic result is that uninsured (and underinsured) individuals are

TABLE 8.1

Making a Difference: The HITE Website

PROBLEM

No comprehensive clearinghouse of information for people with inadequate
  health insurance

SOLUTION

Online searchable directory to connect low-income, uninsured, and underinsured individuals with free and low-cost resources

RESULTS

5,000 resources available at the click of a mouse
10,000 searches conducted in the database per month
1,000 health and social services professionals trained to conduct searches
Hundreds of individuals with direct access to 5,000 resources

struggling unnecessarily to access the services they need because they are
often simply unaware of the wide array of free or low-cost health care options available to them.

This situation changed dramatically with the launching of the Health
Information Tool for Empowerment (HITE)—the first interactive online directory of health and social services specifically for uninsured and underinsured New Yorkers. It was my pleasure to join HITE as program coordinator
of Community Voices in the fall of 2003, and to be part of the team that developed this innovative tool. This chapter describes the birth and evolution of
this innovative program that looked to future and developing technology as
a health promotion tool, and my role in bringing it into the world (table 8.1).

An Idea Is Born

It is no secret that our health care system grows more complex each day.
Health care providers experience firsthand how providing information to
people in a community-based, culturally and linguistically sensitive manner improves people's ability to use health programs and services and
increases compliance. But sometimes it seems that this information is
so difficult to access even for professionals that it might as well be buried
under a rock. In 2002 this notion struck home when Rima Cohen, vice president of the foundation arm of the Greater New York Hospital Association

(GNYHA), a trade organization representing and advocating for hospitals and continuing care organizations, was visiting with social workers in Harlem. She observed that the social workers had to peruse tall stacks of paper binders and make several phone calls to help their clients find the information they needed. Much of the information was there, but it was neither organized nor easily available. And, of course, paper directories become outdated quickly. As a result, it was difficult for the social workers to identify all the national, state, and local programs available to their clients. This was Rima Cohen's "aha moment."

When I asked Cohen about the birth of HITE, she said,

I came up with the concept of developing an online tool to help social service professionals when I was directing a project designed to expand health insurance coverage in New York. In the course of that work, I encountered many people who had no coverage or inadequate coverage and realized that even those individuals who qualify for public health insurance or subsidized private coverage often do not know how to enroll in insurance programs, and often do not know about other free or low-cost support services that are available to them. I realized that there is no central database of information to help these individuals—or the professionals who work with them—navigate New York's complex health and social service safety net system. The idea behind HITE was to put information about all these resources—some of which are very local—in one place.

Shortly after conceiving the idea, Cohen hired an assistant to research the idea and help write grants to obtain funding to turn the concept into a reality. The resulting support from the Robert Wood Johnson, Langeloth, and W. K. Kellogg foundations and others enabled them to research and develop the concept more fully. The Robert Wood Johnson Foundation would also come to fund an outside evaluation of the project.

Like all newborns, the concept needed a name. As Cohen recalls, "It seemed like everything we came up with had already been used. Finally we came up with the 'HITE Network'—the Health Insurance, Training, and Education Network—though no one was fully satisfied with that name. A year or two later we were looking to shorten the name and came up with Health Information Tool for Empowerment (HITE) which came closer to describing the website" and its aims.

Finding the right name was an important accomplishment, but before designing the online social service directory, the GNYHA Foundation had to understand the barriers and concerns about providing direct services to the community. So, the first step was to conduct community research. In early 2003 the foundation conducted several focus groups and surveyed more than two hundred professionals in social service and health care organizations serving low-income populations. Cohen says the research was needed "to confirm my observation that nothing like HITE was available in New York City or in the rest of the state."

The most telling finding of her research was that 50 percent of the participants said the main barrier to providing service was the need to spend thirty minutes to two hours searching for resources for each uninsured client. The most common time-consuming problems workers faced were:

- Too much time was needed to find information.
- They did not know about available resources.
- They did not know where to go for information.

Other challenges that social services agencies constantly faced were:

- There was no system for linking uninsured people with resources.
- Uninsured people have multiple, complex needs.
- Health care providers and caseworkers have limited time and heavy caseloads.
- The startling lack of awareness about available resources, even among experienced workers, was due to reliance on word-of-mouth and out-of-date directories, and loss of institutional memory when workers leave.

These findings were the confirmation that the GNYHA Foundation needed to go forward. Although at the time the foundation knew that obtaining computer and Internet access was going to be a challenge for many community providers, it was also evident that online research was going to be the next big thing. Now the question was: where do we begin? Cohen knew she needed partners to help answer that question and to act as pilot sites, and that the partnership would be a close collaboration:

I was very interested in finding the right community partners for the project and spent many months interviewing community leaders and health care experts across the state, and reviewing responses to the Request for Proposals for "lead community partners." The unique aspect of this project was the level of outreach and consultation with community leaders and representatives of the types of professionals such as social workers, case managers, facilitated enrollers, and uninsured individuals who were our target market for HITE, and our formal partnership with community organizations such as the Northern Manhattan Community Voices Collaborative. We were determined to build something that would be useful to the people who we wanted to use and benefit from HITE, and that we were backed by the credibility of these organizations.

This strategy would prove to be a winning one in promoting use of the site.

The Partners and the Pilot Testing

By the fall of 2003 the GNYHA Foundation contracted with three partners to assist in pilot testing, promoting, and training the users in the site. The three partners were prominent community-based health and social service coalitions: the Northern Manhattan Community Voices Collaborative, which represented central Harlem and Washington Heights/Inwood; the Greater Brooklyn Health Coalition, a consortium of more than sixty organizations committed to improving health care access and services in Brooklyn; and Mothers & Babies Perinatal Network of South Central New York, which represents an extensive coalition of health and social service providers, health care plans, community advocacy organizations, and public agencies throughout a seven-county region in upstate New York. Of the partnership with NMCVC, Cohen says, "It was very clear to me that the NMCVC was the ideal partner for northern Manhattan. The NMCVC was one of three key community partners that helped me and the HITE staff member translate the concept of an online tool for health and social service professionals into a reality. Because it is so well-respected, and because of its connection to important policymakers, professionals, and community residents, Voices gave the HITE project the credibility it needed to succeed in northern Manhattan—one of the target underserved areas that could benefit greatly from HITE."

Following Cohen's visionary leadership as director, each partner played an active role in the development and implementation of HITE. She says, "NMCVC and the two other community-based organizations helped me make many of the key decisions with respect to the web site—including decisions about the site's design, content, navigation, and its 'look and feel.' Voices also played a key role in educating residents and organizations in northern Manhattan about the availability of the tool, and in training these individuals and staff of organizations to use HITE." Each partner also identified key community resources as well as assisting with outreach efforts in the promotion and usage of HITE with their community.

Once the basic website design was completed, the next step was to begin data collection. This was when I joined the NMCVC team. When I first heard about HITE, I was extremely excited to be part of this monumental community project. I knew firsthand the importance of having an online resource tool. Before joining Community Voices, I had worked in the asthma outreach program of a nonprofit organization. Although I was given extensive training and orientation about asthma, I had very little knowledge about the community I was serving. All I was told was that there was a high asthma and absentee rate in my assigned school and that I needed to conduct home visits. I remember the frustration I felt when I wanted to help the parents, but I had no idea where to send them when they needed information unrelated to asthma. While I was building my network and contacts list, at times it seemed like I was trying to knock down brick walls. I went through months of pure frustration. Even though I was making endless phone calls, studying countless directories, attending community meetings, and engaging in numerous ways of networking, I felt I was not getting the information my clients needed. It took six months for me to feel 80 percent confident that I could provide my clients with the appropriate resources and tools. It was through this experience that I knew the value of HITE. And so, I was thrilled to be part of this collaboration.

My job was to assist in data collection. Our catchment area included ten zip codes and stretched from 110th Street to the northern tip of Manhattan and from the Hudson River on the west side to the East River—about a ten-mile radius. We collected information from existing paper-based community resource guides and directories created by local institutions and community-based agencies. These resource guides contained information on programs and services directed to dental and optical services, primary health, mental health, social service organizations, and support for immigrants. Over the course of the next six months, I was part of the team that called them, using a questionnaire created by the HITE staff to guide us in gathering the specific information to be included in the HITE database. To ensure that the database was comprehensive and accurate, NMCVC and HITE staff members made multiple calls to the agencies to verify their information.

We collected data for thousands of resources, ranging from mental and dental health centers to immigrant support services. I cannot describe the great feeling I had once the data was entered and the website content and layout were completed.

The First of Its Kind

What we had created was the first interactive online tool designed specifically to link uninsured and underinsured New Yorkers with a comprehensive directory of the free and low-cost health and social services available to them. Anyone with access to a computer could use the free website—either on their own or with the assistance of health care and social service providers. The HITE website included two main features:

1. A comprehensive, searchable database of national, state, and local health care services and programs for the uninsured and underinsured.
2. Online eligibility calculators to help individuals determine whether they are likely to be eligible for one of New York's public health insurance programs or for a low-cost private insurance program.

HITE users could search for resources by zip code, services offered, medical conditions treated, and languages spoken. The information provided included clinics and other health care facilities, public health insurance programs, free or low-cost prescription drugs, immigrant support services, immunizations or health screenings with a sliding scale fee, free transportation, and hundreds of other programs designed specifically for low-income, uninsured individuals.

Launching HITE

After a year of data collection and modifications in the website content and design, HITE was ready to go live. In the spring of 2005, during "Cover the Uninsured Week," the Greater New York Hospital Foundation and the Northern Manhattan Community Voices Collaborative launched HITE in northern Manhattan. To say this was an exciting moment for the NMCVC would be an understatement. Making the experience all the sweeter was the fact that community Internet research was just then gaining popularity in the social services industry. So, HITE had perfect timing.

The Northern Manhattan Improvement Corporation (NMIC), an NMCVC partner, was the carefully chosen social services organization that kicked off the HITE website. "NMIC has been a haven for thousands of newly immigrant families," said Jacqueline Martínez, executive director of the NMCVC at Columbia University Medical Center. "It was fitting that the HITE initiative was launched in this organization and used to strengthen their role of social service providers in northern Manhattan." Thus, twenty-six NMIC staff members were the first to witness, experience, and be trained on the online tool. By the end of the day, all of the NMIC staff who experienced the one-day HITE training were eager to put it into practice and share the news. María Lizardo, director of social services at NMIC, concluded, "This online tool will make navigating the health care system and wide array of social services so much easier and efficient. Not only will the provider's job be made easier, but our constituents will benefit tremendously from this new online tool."

For the next several months, training and outreach efforts became the NMCVC's central focus to promote HITE to the northern Manhattan community. As we knew would happen, one of our major challenges in promoting and conducting HITE training was the lack of computer laboratory and Internet connections. Undaunted, we still engaged all of our partner organizations and promoted the use of the HITE website through the entire community because we knew that in time most if not all of the agencies would have computer and Internet access for their staff.

Up and Running

By fall 2006 more than thirty agencies—close to two hundred health care providers—in northern Manhattan had received a two-hour HITE training conducted by NMCVC staff. These included health care facilities, clinics, social service agencies, school administration, faith-based organizations, and libraries. Around this time, the New York Academy of Medicine, an independent research, education, and advocacy organization, was contracted to conduct an evaluation of HITE. The researchers emailed surveys to 1,674 users of HITE; of these, 274 complete and usable surveys were returned and analyzed.

The New York Academy of Medicine survey found that the vast majority of respondents, across all user types, agreed that HITE was a useful and effective resource. Nearly all respondents (96%) said they would recommend HITE to a colleague. Respondents who completed the frequent user survey, which posed an additional series of questions about HITE, were particularly enthusiastic about the site. Nearly all frequent users (93%) reported that they were able to serve more people more effectively since they began using HITE, and about half (48%) of these users identified HITE as their main source of information about low-cost health and social services, while 65 percent agreed that they rely less on other sources of information since using HITE. Frequent users also agreed that their clients were able to successfully access services that were identified using HITE (95%).

The report also shed light on who was using the site. The majority of the HITE users were female (82%), college educated (82%), and between the ages of 25 and 44 (58%); nearly half (49%) had graduate degrees. Thirty-five percent of respondents reported using HITE five or more times (frequent users), 40 percent reported using it two to four times (infrequent users), and 25 percent reported using it once or never (nonusers). Nearly half (49%) of the respondents identified as white, 23 percent African American, 21 percent Latino, and 5 percent Asian. Sixty-seven percent reported that their agency provided social work/case management, 36 percent provided medical care, 19 percent administered government programs, and 52 percent provided other kinds of social services (e.g., housing, immigration, legal services).

Still Growing

We knew that the residents of Harlem and Washington Heights/Inwood would benefit greatly from the NMCVC's pioneering efforts, and deployment of the HITE tool to this community further addressed the pressing health care needs of its underserved, uninsured residents. Since HITE's initial pilot test in northern Manhattan, Brooklyn, and the southern tier of New York State, the project received funding to expand to the remaining areas of New York City and Long Island and hopes to expand statewide and eventually nationwide. Clearly, this is only the beginning of a powerful tool.

In the meantime, HITE continues to be an important and growing resource for northern Manhattan. According to Jenne Russo, the current project manager, health and social services professionals representing over a thousand organizations access HITE each month in addition to hundreds of individuals directly seeking care. Nearly ten thousand searches are conducted in the database per month. By mid-2009 HITE staff had trained over a thousand professionals at organizations throughout New York City and Long Island. HITE continued to offer trainings as part of a new outreach initiative in 2009. To keep the information as current and accurate as possible, all of the nearly five thousand resources are updated yearly on a rolling basis. The HITE staff makes phone calls to listed organizations to verify the information, and the site encourages users to review their own organizations' HITE listings as well.

In addition, in 2007 HITE partnered with the city's 311 Call Center system.1 As a result of this partnership, the city's 311 Call Center has expanded its coverage to include information and referrals to local nonprofit health and human service agencies such as social service providers, food pantries, and health centers. Former HITE director Rima Cohen states, "The city of New York is buying HITE's data to use as part of its expanded 311 initiative. This will ensure that millions of individuals who use the city's 311 system every year will have access to HITE's up-to-date, quality, comprehensive information."

Like any other pioneering project, HITE faced many challenges. The main challenge was overcoming the reality that, at the time of its inception, many of the potential users did not have ready access to the Internet. Thanks to a visionary like Rima Cohen and a devoted team who understood the need and saw beyond the norm, today the Health Information Tool for Empowerment has lived up to its name. As computers and the Internet have become ubiquitous in community organizations, homes, and libraries, HITE has heightened and empowered access to better health care and proved to be the blessing we hoped it would be, as the satisfied users sampled in box 8.1 attest.

152

Strengthening the Safety Net

BOX 8.1

Empowerment via the Internet

"This site is so important. I have helped numerous people to find clinics, doctors, and mental health facilities. . . . I am continuously researching questions from people who are in dire need of health care. There are people who are working without green cards and feel they cannot get health care. In confidential interviews, they ask me not to take their names or their children's name just to please to give them some health related information. There are so many needy people, who confidentially come to me with health related questions for service. By myself I really don't know what to do . . . however . . . I find this website to be a useful tool."

"Today [HITE] was a lifesaver. I had a patient (uninsured, undocumented— very sick with cancer). He needed desperately to see a dermatologist. I was able to identify a dermatology clinic in Brooklyn for just $25. I call that miraculous. Thanks for helping me do my job better."

"I use it both to find social services and for the eligibility calculator and I love it. I am a case manager and I train other case managers. HITE is one of the first resources I teach them!"

"As a vocational counselor in a training program, part of my job is to assist students with finding internships in a social service setting. HITE has been a valuable resource for my students, since it locates agencies dealing with the particular population they want to work with, whom they can contact."

Using HITE, consumers can save time and search independently, and caseworkers can be more efficient and less frustrated in providing the best access to care for their clients and patients. And in doing so, health care providers and community organizations are better equipped to reduce health disparities and increase health care access for the million of uninsured and underserved communities.

Northern Manhattan Community Voices Collaborative believed the HITE online tool was a groundbreaking, needed investment—an ideal vehicle for the collaborative to use technology to advance its objectives in increasing access to care among the northern Manhattan community. Much of the impetus for the collaborative's creation came from a pressing need to centralize and coordinate health care promotion and community outreach initiatives, and this was at the core of the HITE mission. Having a central location to access resources was a dream come true, especially for health workers like me who had little or no knowledge of the community in which they were working. We have found that HITE is one avenue, one powerful tool to empower and strengthen underserved communities— and instead of struggling with mountains of paper directories, it is just a click away at www.hitesite.org.

Note

1. In March 2003 the New York City began a new era of government service with the launch of the NYC 311 Citizen Service Center. People dial 311 (or 212-NEW YORK) to reach the service. The 311 project responds to calls from residents, businesses, and visitors by providing reliable information and accurately processing requests for city services twenty-four hours a day, seven days a week.

References

Bishop, A. P., T. J. Tidlinea, S. Shoemaker, and P. Salelaa (1999). Public libraries and networked information services in low-income communities. *Library & Information Science Research* 21, no. 3: 361–90.

Kind, T., Z. Huang, D. Farr, and K. Pomerantz (2005). Internet and computer access and use for health information in an underserved community. *Ambulatory Pediatrics* 5, no. 2: 117–21.

New York Academy of Medicine, Division of Health Policy (2006). *Evaluation of the Health Information Tool for Empowerment (HITE) Network.* http://www.rwjf.org/reports/grr/041710.htm.

New York City Department of Health and Mental Hygiene (2004). *Community survey.* New York: Department of Health and Mental Hygiene.

—— (2006). *Community health profiles.* http://www.nyc.gov/html/doh/html/data/data.shtml.

U.S. Census Bureau (2000). Census data. Washington, D.C.: U.S. Census Bureau.

Selected Additional References

Cover the Uninsured Program website. http://www.covertheuninsured.org.

Health Resources and Services Administration website. http://www.hrsa.gov/ (for information on manpower shortage areas).

Lee, R. C. (1974). Designation of Health Manpower Shortage Areas for use by public health service programs. *Association of Schools of Public Health* 94, no. 1: 48–59.

[9]

HealthGap and the NMCVC's
Effort to Cover the Uninsured

HARRIS K. (KEN) LAMPERT

> Now came the really difficult part—figuring out how much this would
> all cost. . . . This debate brought home for people how difficult it is
> to create an "affordable" insurance plan. Unless you compromise and
> leave some benefits out, there will be no way it will be "affordable."

In the spring of 1998, I got a call from Allan J. Formicola, then the dean of
the Columbia University College of Dental Medicine, formerly known as
the School of Dental and Oral Surgery. He wanted to know if Community
Premier Plus, the tiny, not-for-profit managed care health plan that I was
in charge of, wanted to participate in a grant application to the W. K. Kellogg Foundation for something called "Community Voices." There was not
much time to think about it, as is so often the case with such opportunities, since the application was due within a few months. To be perfectly
honest, I was a bit taken aback—although we were a startup with an entrepreneurial spirit and a commitment to improving the health of the community, our plan had only started serving members in June 1997. Like
most such organizations, the staff was just trying to survive month to
month, grow the business, and learn our way around the world of publicly
funded health insurance.

Looking back, Formicola says he tapped Community Premier Plus to
develop a new health care insurance product "precisely because" we were
"a start up with an entrepreneurial spirit and a commitment to improving
the health of the community." He says, "We realized the myriad of issues
that would need to be thought out would take entrepreneurship and a fresh

approach from a group not tainted by previous attempts. Ken Lampert, a recognized individual, thought analytically and approached tough issues with thoroughness, ideal leadership traits to head up the Health Gap project."

Formicola piqued my interest when he explained the underlying issues that seemed to be driving the W. K. Kellogg Foundation's willingness to invest in our community. He talked about engaging the community in planning for change in the health care system, about pushing for changes in that system that would help it to better meet the needs of those who were medically underserved, and about reducing and eliminating racial and ethnic health disparities. All of this was consistent with the role those of us at Community Premier Plus saw for our health plan. But what really caught my ear was the goal of increasing health insurance coverage for the uninsured. This went to the core of Community Premier Plus's mission. So without really knowing what I was getting myself or my organization into, I signed on. As it turned out, our collaboration with the Northern Manhattan Community Voices Collaborative and the other partners played a critical role in the tremendous growth we achieved in the years that followed and the place we earned as one of the top-rated health plans in New York. Although the product we designed was never implemented, the journey we took to get there serves as an informative cautionary tale to others with goals similar to ours.

TABLE 9.1

Making a Difference: HealthGap Insurance Plan

PROBLEM

Many uninsured individuals not eligible to be covered by existing health plans such as Child Health Plus and Medicaid—a "health gap"

SOLUTION

Design a model health insurance plan for small business, their employees, their spouses, self-employed workers, their spouses, and possibly other adults, with income less than 200 percent of the federal poverty limit

RESULTS

A fairly comprehensive benefit package with an average weighted annual premium of over $2,300 per year for an individual

Community Premier Plus

Community Premier Plus was a somewhat unusual enterprise: a not-for-profit health plan that was owned, governed by, and closely affiliated with big hospital systems, but independently operated and community based. It was licensed as a "prepaid health services plan," a special purpose managed care organization, in 1996 as a result of the collaboration of three of the most important providers of health care to the communities that make up northern Manhattan: Presbyterian Hospital (which later became New York Presbyterian Hospital following a merger), North General Hospital, and Harlem Hospital Center of the New York City Health and Hospitals Corporation. Community Premier Plus was a unique public–private partnership that came about as a result of the state's goal to mandate membership in a managed care health plan for the vast majority of recipients of Medicaid, the federal-state health insurance program for the poorest members of society. The founding hospitals, which relied (and still rely) heavily on revenues from Medicaid, were concerned that they might lose many of their Medicaid patients to other institutions that themselves were the owners of Medicaid managed care companies. The drive for managed care was also driven by the realization on the part of the state and policy experts that something needed to be done to drastically improve on many of Medicaid's flaws—the lack of primary care and prevention, the lack of continuity of care, an overreliance on emergency rooms, a shortage of quality providers willing to accept Medicaid's low fees, and a lack of accountability for quality of care.

Community Premier Plus was incorporated in July 1996, with a board of directors made up of representatives of the three sponsoring hospitals and health plan enrollees. Child Health Plus and Family Health Plus, two new insurance programs for the uninsured, were soon added to the product lineup. Providers were eventually added in the Bronx, which allowed us to broaden our marketing and enrollment efforts beyond Manhattan.

The first twenty members joined in June 1997. The plan grew steadily, eventually enrolling over seventy-five thousand members by 2005. The provider network included primary care providers and specialists affiliated with the three sponsoring institutions as well as private and small group providers with offices in the service area. These community-based providers served a substantial proportion of the enrollees. Community Premier Plus was recognized by the state as one of the top-performing health plans, especially for its customer service and the positive recommendation of the members.

The Problem: A Growing Health Gap

The core issue that drove this aspect of the Community Voices effort was the lack of affordable health insurance for large numbers of New Yorkers, particularly the working poor, small business owners and their employees, and undocumented residents. The implications of this lack of health care coverage for health status have been well documented. The causes of the lack of affordable health coverage are quite complex and rooted in the history of how health care is delivered and paid for in this country. Most Americans are covered through employment-based private insurance; many others are covered through government programs such as Medicare and Medicaid. But these approaches leave large gaps through which tens of millions have fallen. The idea behind the Community Voices insurance effort was to help fill some of those gaps in the insurance safety net—hence we coined the term "HealthGap" for the product we envisioned. Simply put, at the onset of the grant, the NMCVC and the W. K. Kellogg Foundation wanted Community Premier Plus to aim for a new insurance product that was geared to the needs of the uninsured parents of Child Health Plus enrollees and small business owners.

Initial Research

Right after the Kellogg Foundation awarded the grant to Community Voices, we got down to work. First and foremost, we needed to make sure we understood the needs of the community and that we had input from all of the stakeholders. So, we formed a working group, the process favored by the NMCVC for bringing various voices to the table and for planning on how to address the problem. The resulting Insurance Product working group was cochaired by me and Stephen Marshall, from the Columbia College of Dental Medicine. The idea was not that everyone was an expert in health insurance, but rather that the members represented a cross-section of academia, businesses, and community-based organizations. The working group was intended to guide the overall direction of the project. Unfortunately, the group never really seemed to gel. We realized that part of the problem was the highly technical nature of the development of this product. While the working group was able to come up with broad goals, the actual development of an insurance product would take the expertise of Community Premier Plus and outside consultants. Over time the working group sort of faded away, and direction for the program was given by the NMCVC leadership.

Before we took the next big step of designing a product that would meet the needs of the community, we needed to learn more about the population we wanted to serve. For starters, we had to learn much more about the specific causes of lack of insurance coverage and the concerns within the varied communities served by Community Voices and Community Premier Plus. We needed to understand what kinds of solutions would make sense to the community. This went to one of the core goals of Community Voices— to engage the community in dialogue and get input about the problems and the potential solutions. It was not enough for us to "deliver" a health insurance product, assuming we could pull that off—it had to be relevant to the actual needs and perceptions of the people it was intended to help. It also had to have buy-in from community-based organizations that would be expected to recommend it and, most critically, the health care providers who would be paid by Community Premier Plus for providing services to the newly insured beneficiaries of this innovative health insurance product. As we started to look more carefully at the issues, we at Community Premier Plus became concerned that the creation of a new insurance product would be very difficult. But we felt strongly that we needed to learn all we could about the problem of lack of affordable health insurance in the communities we served—the numbers of the uninsured, who was in this group, the depth of knowledge that individuals had about health insurance, and the impact of not having insurance on their lives.

So, our next step was to survey the community. In 2000 we conducted surveys of small business owners and their employees, livery cab drivers (who are self-employed), street vendors, and small business customers in Washington Heights and Harlem. We asked whether they had health insurance and, if they did not have it, how this impacted them. We also asked about emergency room use. Finally, we asked them what benefits they wanted the most in an affordable insurance product.

As a result of the community survey, we learned that the small business owners—and these were very small, mostly retail establishments (such as

bodegas and beauty salons), with an average of three or four employees—
were not very interested in covering their employees. Although they were
not especially conversant in insurance matters, they were interested in
coverage for themselves and family members. The top priorities for benefits were doctor's visits and hospitalization, followed by dental care and
prescription drugs. Only 30 percent of the individuals surveyed had visited
an emergency room in the past year. Many had paid out-of-pocket for
checkups and other medical care. The small business environment was of
particular interest, given the fact that these types of businesses are the
least likely to offer employer-sponsored health coverage, and the importance assigned to them in the original NMCVC assessment of the focus
population for HealthGap. We learned that 43 percent of the 6,982 businesses in upper Manhattan in the 1997 census had fewer than five employees; only 2–6% had more than fifty employees. All of these data indicated
that marketing a new product in this environment could turn out to be
extremely costly and slow.

Considering the Climate at the Time

We also needed a clear understanding of the regulatory, financial, and programmatic challenges that would be faced by a small plan such as Community Premier Plus operating in a very complex, competitive, and highly
regulated environment. One of the things that was not well established
from the outset was buy-in from Community Premier Plus's sponsoring
hospitals, especially in light of existing mechanisms, such as emergency
Medicaid and the state bad debt and charity care pools, that paid for at least
some of the care they provided to the uninsured. It was by no means certain that they would support such a product, especially if it might put any
of this well-established funding at risk.

At the same time as we were conducting our research, the New York
State government was already moving toward new solutions for uninsured
populations. There was an emerging bipartisan consensus that something
had to be done without waiting for the federal government to take action.
As a result, several new state-funded or subsidized programs were developed for low-income people, the working poor, and small businesses left
out of the commercial market: the Child Health Plus program, which under-
went a major expansion in December 1997; Family Health Plus, a program

for people with income above the Medicaid limits, which started enrollment in 2002; and Healthy New York, a reduced-cost benefit package sold
by health maintenance organizations to small businesses and the self-
employed. In addition, facilitated enrollment became a reality in 2002 as
well. Facilitated enrollment, unique to New York State, is a process that allows the government to delegate to community-based organizations and
health plans such as Community Premier Plus a lead role in much of the
enrollment process for publicly funded health care, especially the mandatory face-to-face interview. Ultimately both Community Premier Plus and
Alianza Dominicana, another NMCVC collaborator, became certified as facilitated enrollers (see chapter 3 for this story). In light of this rapidly changing environment, it became critical to keep abreast of these changes—
both as a core responsibility of Community Premier Plus and for the
success of the NMCVC endeavor as well.

With the help of a graduate student from the Columbia University Mailman School of Public Health, Michael Resnick, and his mentor Sherry
Glied, professor of health policy and management, we started to learn
more about the demographic makeup of the communities we intended to
serve—especially how many eligible uninsured there might be. This was
obviously a key question, but one that was not easy to answer. To do this,
Michael used databases such as the Current Population Survey and census
data. He also helped us try to understand how other funding streams for
the care of the uninsured, such as the Bad Debt and Charity Care Health
Care Reform Act pools, were supposed to work. This is a pretty arcane and
complex subject, but we felt we had to understand the environment in
which the hospitals and other providers worked—and whether they would
be receptive to a change in how they were paid for the care provided to at
least some of the uninsured who relied on them.

Designing the Product

We then took what we learned, discussed it with the working group and
others in the community, and started to put together our model insurance
product. Once we had our benefit design and our assumptions on enrollment, demographics, and pricing (based on Community Premier Plus's
existing provider contracts), we hired a certified actuary to price out our
proposal (see below). We also started to think about the program features

for HealthGap and how we might market it. Along the way we presented our ideas at a meeting with the United Hospital Fund, at which other community-based insurance program representatives discussed what they were trying to accomplish. This gave us a lot of useful feedback from others who were also struggling to implement innovative insurance solutions. Although several Community Premier Plus staff members and outside consultants reworked this initial version over the next five years, the core concepts remained.

Early on we established eight program goals:

- affordable and accessible insurance coverage for the uninsured population
- a program that would meet the needs of small businesses, their employees, and the self-employed in a low-income community
- improved individual health status through an emphasis on preventive care
- prevention of economic dislocation due to catastrophic illness
- improved public health in a community already confronting poor health status due to preventable and treatable conditions
- financial support for safety net providers
- reduced state expenditures on emergency Medicaid
- ease of enrollment and program sustainability

Eligibility was going to be restricted to persons who could not qualify for existing programs—thus filling the "health coverage gap." Enrollment would be limited to owners and employees of small businesses (fewer than fifty employees), self-employed workers, their spouses, and possibly people who resided in but did not work in the service area, defined as twelve zip codes in northern Manhattan. (Children were not included because, as a result of existing program rules and a state court decision, all children, including the undocumented, were eligible for Child Health Plus.) Family income would have to be equal to or less than 200 percent of the federal poverty limit; age must be between 19 and 64; the applicant could not have voluntarily canceled employment-based insurance; and the applicant must be screened for and found to be ineligible for Medicaid and Family Health Plus.

The benefit package was quite comprehensive, including primary and preventive care, hospitalization for both physical and mental disorders as well as substance abuse, outpatient surgery, professional fees, diagnostic testing, outpatient chemotherapy and radiation therapy, maternity care, home health care, emergency room services, nutritional counseling, diabetes education and supplies, outpatient mental health and substance abuse treatment, and pharmacy benefits up to $2,500 per year. Services such as long-term care, hospice, cosmetic procedures, nonemergency transportation and personal care services were excluded from the benefit package. One of the issues we debated with the working group was whether or not we should include dental benefits. This added considerably to the costs, which we were trying to keep down, but of course it was a tough sell not to include them given the great need for these services, the priority given to this in our community surveys, and the close involvement in the NMCVC of the Columbia College of Dental Medicine. After all, Allan Formicola, as the dean of the dental school, was the leader of Community Voices! But this debate brought home for people how difficult it is to create an affordable insurance plan. Unless you compromise and leave some benefits out, there will be no way it will be affordable. Although we initially left out dental coverage, it was eventually added back in.

One of the major approaches to keeping down the premium costs was to require copays for most services, ranging from $15 for an office visit to $750 per hospital stay to $20 for a generic prescription. This was controversial, as there had always been a concern that copays and coinsurance would create financial barriers to care for low-income recipients of publicly funded insurance. But as difficult as it would be to get state support for this program, it would be nearly impossible without requiring some degree of "taking responsibility" by the recipients. This was a core part of many of the new programs supported by the Pataki administration, especially Healthy New York.

Now came the really difficult part—figuring out how much this would all cost. To answer that critical question, we gave the benefit package and a projection of how many people (and the age/income/sex breakdown of this potential group of enrollees) would take up coverage to Edward Kumian at Interpretive Data Specialists. Their actuaries used industry-standard assumptions on the characteristics of an uninsured population getting coverage for the first time (including their rates of utilization and the impact of the copays), as well as Community Premier Plus's contracted rates with our provider network. (For the sake of making the premiums as low as possible, we had discounted some of those rates by 25 percent.) They also built in trend factors for changes in utilization and costs and an added factor for administrative costs. They broke the population down into six actuarial categories based on age and sex. In addition to the medical and administrative costs, they had to build in state-mandated Health Care Reform Act taxes and assessments that would almost certainly apply to a product such as HealthGap.

Table 9.2 shows the initial rates without dental coverage, just to give an idea of what such coverage would have cost in 2001. It would surely be much more now.

When we decided to add dental benefits, an additional $13–14 per member per month was added to the final rate. We also put forth several suggestions as to how these rates could be brought down further, such as elimination of some benefits, bigger discounts from providers (although hospital rates had already been discounted by 25 percent to get to these premiums), grant support for marketing and outreach activities, state-provided reinsurance protection (as was the case for Healthy New York), and a waiver of Health Care Reform Act taxes and assessments. Unfortunately, most of these were either unpalatable or impractical.

With an average weighted premium of $193 (based on the expected mix of age and sex categories), if we had ended the first year with 1,200 enrollees and had grown to 3,500 by the end of the third year, we would have needed over $13 million in premium revenue annually. Since we felt it would be impossible to get these low-income enrollees to pay the full premiums—and, based on previous experience with Child Health Plus, it

TABLE 9.2

Initial Premiums Rates

RATE	CATEGORY	BASE MEDICAL	HCRA TAX AND COVERED LIFE ASSESSMENT	ADMINISTRATION AND REINSURANCE	FINAL RATE
19–29	Male	$81.17	11.73	14.74	107.64
19–29	Female	139.88	16.08	24.20	180.16
30–44	Male	158.80	16.32	27.07	202.19
30–44	Female	141.01	15.44	24.27	180.72
45–64	Male	257.51	22.49	42.81	322.81
45–64	Female	248.68	22.13	41.43	312.24

would be very difficult to collect even a minimal member contribution—
we agreed that we would need the state to subsidize the entire cost.

Finally, to make this work we would need a robust advocacy strategy
with the state legislature and the departments of health and insurance,
an evaluation component, and creative and cost-saving ways to market the
program and enroll people who had little or no experience with navigating
the world of health coverage.

Results

We introduced the first version of HealthGap in July 2001, three years after
the beginning of the W. K. Kellogg Foundation grant. We spent the next
few years fine-tuning the proposal and trying to figure out ways to get it
funded. Figuring out how this would be paid for was the most difficult
part of the project. The goal had never been just to write a nice paper that
would sit on the shelf, although we were very pleased that we had the opportunity to present what we learned at various Kellogg Foundation national forums, including a Community Voices meeting in Miami in 2005.
HealthGap was also written up and compared with the results of the other
Community Voices projects in a 2005 report by the Economic & Social
Research Institute.

But the simple fact was that we were up against a seemingly insurmountable barrier: the lack of any funding stream to pay for the premiums.
The whole project had been predicated on the notion that at best we could
get the enrollees to pay copays when they received care. We would never be
able to get them to pay $13 million in premiums—that burden would have
to be borne by the state. (And what would happen after the initial three
years? We never got close to discussing sustainability.) But there were no
state Requests for Proposals out there for new insurance models, and we
did not have enough clout to get special legislation passed that would provide such a large amount of money benefiting only one community in the
state. (One of the aspects of Community Voices that never took off, despite
much discussion, was a legislative and lobbying strategy to support this and
other initiatives. It was not Community Premier Plus's role, especially as a
government contractor, to be the prime actor in this.) In fact, there were
many new initiatives coming on line, as noted earlier—Family Health Plus,

the expansion of Child Health Plus, and Healthy New York—that, combined with the dire economic circumstances following the September 2001 attack on the World Trade Center, made it highly unlikely that a new funding stream would open up. There was no program or initiative that we could latch onto to get traction for funding of HealthGap. Although there was ongoing dialogue with Community Voices about these issues, there was not a decision-making process that brought us to this point—the reality of the situation spoke for itself.

When that became clear, we increasingly focused our time and energy on marketing and building up enrollment in programs such as Family Health Plus, which, through the efforts of many health plans, community-based organizations, and county social service agencies, eventually brought health coverage to over a half million New Yorkers. There were further efforts made to refine the HealthGap model and rewrite the paper to make it more of a think piece, but Community Premier Plus mostly focused on bringing services and coverage to the community through the existing lines of business and planning for new initiatives such as Medicare managed care. When the original grant ended after five years, Community Premier Plus retained its connection to the ongoing Community Voices initiative, but unfortunately HealthGap ended up, as we had feared, on the shelf.

Lessons Learned

So much work went into HealthGap; although it was very frustrating not to be able to offer it and test out our ideas—and to actually provide insurance coverage to those who had gone without much health care for so many years—we did learn quite a bit. We learned a lot about the problems of the uninsured in the communities we served and the difficulties encountered in trying to solve this problem. The core problems were beyond the scope of this project, even if we had been successful in launching a pilot product. To begin with, health care in the United States is very expensive and getting more expensive all the time, even for a normal-risk population that has been receiving regular health care. Uninsured people, and especially poor people and recent immigrants, have significant unmet health care needs that must be taken care of when they join a health plan. Any plan that covers them must be prepared to play catch-up—which adds considerably to costs. All discussions about "affordable" insurance and "affordable" health care are relative—there is no such thing as inexpensive, high-quality health care. We were a not-for-profit, and we were prepared to ask our hospital providers to take a 25 percent discount off of Medicaid inpatient rates. Even with this and copays, the average weighted premium for a fairly comprehensive benefit package was going to be over $2,300 per year for an individual.

In many ways it was quite a leap for a plan our size to take this on. Even the largest insurers, with the ability to spread their overhead over hundreds of thousands or millions of premium-paying covered lives, would think twice about pursuing this, at least not without the guarantee of state support. Even a program such as Healthy New York, with significant support from the governor and financial protection against major losses by the insurers, was very slow to take off in the early years.

The problem of the uninsured is a national one, closely connected to the fate of the safety net providers who are left with the burden of caring for them. The history of the past fifteen years since the Clinton health reform fizzled as well as the 2008 presidential campaign illustrate very well the difficulty in addressing these issues—and the enormous sums of money that one way or another will be required. The from-the-ground-up, community-empowerment model that to my mind underlay the approach pursued by the W. K. Kellogg Foundation can and should be a very important part of the search for state and national solutions to this problem. But even with grant funding, it is a stretch for a small community-based organization such as Community Premier Plus to have much of an impact. All of our time and energy was committed to building our Medicaid, Family Health Plus, and Child Health Plus lines of business, while partnering with our providers to improve the quality of care for our members. This is especially the case in an urban environment such as New York City, where there are so many competing interests and complex relationships between government units and the funding streams they control, health care providers, other insurance companies, and various segments of the public.

I would advise any organization such as Community Premier Plus to be both cautious and bold when confronted with this kind of opportunity—cautious in that one has to be realistic about what a small organization can accomplish in the face of such difficult odds, and bold in that someone has to step forward and test out new approaches. But perhaps all of us in Community Voices—and the community we were committed to—would have been better served if the resources that the grant put at our disposal had gone into reaching more of the thousands of eligible uninsured and getting them into existing coverage programs. We could have also pushed more forcefully for Community Voices to become a vocal advocate in the public arena for expansions of those programs so that even more of the uninsured could become eligible. HealthGap in some ways was a bit of a distraction from the core problems, and even if enacted it would have touched the lives of only a tiny minority of the uninsured.

In many ways the NMCVC experience brought Community Premier Plus closer to the communities we served and to many organizations and people who in the end were very supportive of our work. It brought a whole new dimension to our mission—not just that we would work within the structures laid down by the state and city for publicly funded managed care plans, but that we could conceive of creating something totally new that was tailored to meet the needs of the community. We were all grateful for that opportunity.

References

Committee on the Consequences of Uninsurance, Board on Health Care Services, Institute of Medicine (2002). *Care without coverage: Too little, too late.* Washington, D.C.: National Academy Press.

New York City Department of Health and Mental Hygiene (2000). *2000 census profiles for New York City.* http://gis.nyc.gov/dcp/pa/address.jsp.

New York State Department of Health (2008). *Healthy New York.* http://www.ins.state.ny.us/website2/hny/english/hnyfhch.htm.

Silow-Carroll, S., and T. Alteras (2005). *Community-based health coverage programs: Models and lessons.* Economic and Social Research Institute, May.

Silow-Carroll, S., T. Alteras, and L. Stepnick (2006). Patient-centered care for underserved populations: Definition and best practices. *Economic and Social Research Institute*: 1–43.

10

Healthy Choices

Mobilizing Community Assets to Combat the Twin Epidemic of Obesity and Diabetes

JACQUELINE MARTÍNEZ and YISEL ALONZO

> Like tobacco control, the obesity and diabetes crisis had given the pub-
> lic health field an opportunity to reclaim its historic role as a change
> agent focused on the environment and public policy.

The obesity and diabetes epidemics are among the most serious public
health threats facing communities across the United States. Over the past
four decades U.S. obesity rates have nearly quadrupled to over 30 percent,
and type 2 diabetes rates have grown from 5.2 percent in 1980 to more than
8 percent of the population. Today, approximately 20 million Americans
have type II diabetes, and another 54 million more have prediabetes, putting
them at high risk for developing the disease. Nearly 25 million children and
adolescents are overweight or obese. In addition, more than 75,000 individuals under age 20 have diabetes, and 2 million aged 12–19 have prediabetes.
In New York City, overall nearly one person in eight has diabetes. However,
the risk is not evenly distributed; for example, the prevalence among Latinos
under age 40 is 3 percent, which is twice that of African Americans and four
times that of non-Latino whites and Asians.

The strain on the economy, in terms of health care costs and loss of pro-
ductivity associated with these two conditions, has already reached crisis
proportions. Diabetes and obesity are causing a severe financial drain on our
health care system. According to the Department of Health and Human
Services, obese and overweight adults cost the United States anywhere from
$69 billion to $117 billion per year. Childhood obesity alone is estimated to
cost the nation up to $14 billion each year in direct health care costs.

The United States has arrived at this juncture because of a nexus of environmental and social trends. Nearly a third of children and teens eat fast food at least once a day; adults consume larger portions of more unhealthy, processed foods; school-aged kids spend more than four nonschool hours in front of a screen; nine out of ten kids are driven to school versus biking or walking. But it is clear that the underlying causes of these behavioral trends are rooted in factors beyond individual control. Several of the main contributing factors to obesity include the high cost of healthful foods, lack of grocery stores, disproportionate numbers of fast-food restaurants located in low-income neighborhoods, poor access to safe places to exercise, and the unavailability of preventive health care services. Therefore reversing the diabetes and obesity epidemics will call for multiple-level interventions at the community and policy levels to effect change in the physical and social environment, including making healthy eating options more accessible and restoring physical activities as a routine part of life.

These statistics and, more important, the underlying issues of social and environmental inequities were the driving force behind the decision and commitment of the North Manhattan Community Voices Collaborative's Health Promotion and Disease Prevention working group to tackle this issue. In this chapter, Jacqueline Martínez and Yisel Alonzo write about the efforts of that commitment—the Healthy Choices program, a local initiative that was developed to engage community members and leaders in addressing the immediate and long-term public health problems associated with diabetes and obesity. Both of them worked on the project with a passion that grew out of their professional and personal experiences with the reality of social and economic determinants of health relating to weight struggles and diabetes. Jacqueline Martínez was executive director of the NMCVC and also headed up the HP/DP working group responsible for the Healthy Choices program. Yisel Alonzo, Community Voices program coordinator, came onboard after the program had been launched to help implement it and keep it going. Although it did not achieve the large-scale impact that was intended, the program illustrates the level of concern and commitment on the part of the residents affected by the twin epidemics, and it left behind a product—a curriculum for healthier living—that represents the distillation of what was learned as a result of the program. Like tobacco control, the obesity and diabetes crisis has given the public health field an opportunity to reclaim its historic role as a change agent focused on the environment and public policy.

Developing a Strategy for Change: Identifying Challenges and Champions While Linking Resources

The Health Promotion and Disease Prevention working group was in this for the long haul—we did not want to create another program that began with great fanfare and, after a few months of activity, left few if any lasting changes. We realized we would need to support people's commitment to change their lifestyles permanently. We also knew that any enduring reversal of the obesity and diabetes epidemics must take into account not only a lack of recreational activity and safe space and an unfriendly environment to healthy nutrition, but also how these factors are confounded by increasing economic instability, wavering job security, deteriorating housing conditions, and other chronic conditions, like asthma and depression. It was clear to the staff of Northern Manhattan Community Voices that a by-product of the social and environmental conditions, and a precursor to high-risk behavior, is the level of physical and emotional stress endured in these communities. (These conditions are described in detail in chapter 3.)

It was critical for us to understand the framework of the problem and identify the resources that would go beyond addressing one health problem at a time. Instead of allowing turbulent times to permanently dismantle these communities, the residents of northern Manhattan joined with organizations like Alianza Dominicana, the Northern Manhattan Improvement Corporation, Fresh Youth Initiatives, the Harlem Children's Zone, the Northern Manhattan Perinatal Partnership, the Dominican Women's Development Center, and the Morningside Area Alliance, among many others, which began to emerge in the 1980s and 1990s and collectively began to raise their voices and fight the destruction of their neighborhoods. Such was the backdrop for Community Voices' aim to address concerns related to obesity and diabetes. Our HP/DP working group sought to build on the strengths and assets of these neighborhoods and continue to advance the leadership that had already emerged.

Our key strategy was to facilitate linkages between existing organizations and programs that aimed to empower families and youth and served the immediate needs of the community. There were three sectors we sought to influence and connect: community-based organizations (neighborhood), schools (families and youth), and health and academic institutions (providers and educators). The strategy was to connect these three sectors and enhance existing resources by building mutually beneficial partnerships without adding unnecessary strain or burden on any of them. Our ultimate goal was to create a network of services that led to increased opportunities for physical activity, access to healthier food choices, and community-based screening and prevention efforts. More so, Community Voices staff members sought to identify the people who would serve as agents of change within existing organizations to develop local solutions for healthy eating and routine physical activity. As leaders of the HP/DP working group, we needed to activate the issue of obesity and diabetes among local leaders and build consensus on the necessary steps to tackle the problem.

Assessing Local Assets and Needs

As with any well-designed pubic health initiative, we really needed to know more about the community we sought to work in. Throughout the decade of the 1990s, the Centers for Disease Control continued to paint a clearer picture of the increasing rates of obesity and diabetes across the United States. The data and the increasing trends mentioned earlier in this chapter were very disturbing. However, what we did not know was how northern Manhattan compared in terms of prevalence of these conditions. (Today, the New York City Department of Health and Mental Hygiene publishes *Community Health Profiles*; there was no such data resource during the initial development of the NMCVC.) We also wanted to know whether the obesity and diabetes rates were a priority concern for northern Manhattan residents. Was there already a sense of urgency among the leadership?

The members of the HP/DP working group invested much of their time in the early months to devise a plan to answer some, if not all, of these important questions. The plan included the staff of Community Voices working together with faculty members from the School of Public Health and the leadership of Alianza Dominicana to design a survey to assess the needs of the community as perceived by residents of northern Manhattan. (See chapter 2 for more about the survey, conducted in 1998–1999.) At the end of the needs assessment process, ten priority health problems emerged; exercise, nutrition, and diabetes were among the top five. Over 36 percent of community-based organizations and 34 percent of the population surveyed emphasized that diabetes was their major concern. In addition, community residents indicated a strong desire to lose weight by increasing physical activity and learning more about proper diets for healthy nutrition. We also gathered data through informal discussions with groups of parents in local high schools and school staff. They too indicated that there was a substantial interest in an opportunity to be physically active and for nutrition education.

In the fall of 1999, around the same time the HP/DP survey results were obtained, Columbia University's Mailman School of Public Health administered another survey to school-based health clinics in three elementary and three high schools in northern Manhattan to examine the prevalence of obesity among students. In addition to asking questions about obesity and measuring body-mass index (BMI, a measure of healthy weight), the survey also asked students, parents, and school administrations how they felt about nutrition and physical activity in their community. The survey sample included 2,271 children and adolescents, along with more than 50 parents and teachers at a local high school. The information that resulted indicated a relatively high rate of obesity among males and females: Over 25 percent of the students surveyed were diagnosed as obese—or about 6 percent higher than the national average. The survey also revealed that 90 percent of the adolescents classified as obese were aware they needed to lose weight, and only 10 percent thought they were just the right weight. Nearly all of them indicated a high interest in participating in activities that would allow them to become physically fit.

Our research clearly indicated that increasing community awareness of the problem was not necessary. The numbers of lives affected by obesity, diabetes, and heart conditions had already created a sense of urgency among residents of northern Manhattan. The real question on the table was: what do we do about it?

The Nutrition and Wellness Initiative

As a result of these surveys, the HP/DP working group proposed a Nutrition and Wellness Initiative to the NMCVC executive committee and steering committee. Like the other Community Voices initiatives, our staff and members of the collaborative believed that any program should draw upon existing resources; create strong linkages across community-based initiatives, citywide programs, and health care and education institutions; and increase the effectiveness of the resources already available. We also needed to figure out how we would channel the leadership of the community to focus attention on the environmental policies that needed to change in order to have a safer and nutritionally healthier community. Members of the working group also felt strongly that the city and local government should play an integral role in funding health promotion and disease prevention programs that would increase opportunities for physical activity and healthier diets.

So how did we go about it? For our infrastructure, the HP/DP working group formed a Nutrition and Wellness subcommittee. This was comprised of fifteen organizations and twenty individual members with a common goal: increase the effectiveness of resources available and increase opportunities for optimal nutrition and physical exercise. At the time, there was one program coordinator for this working group and for the four other high-priority areas (asthma, childhood immunization, tobacco cessation, and emergency room reduction) that were still under development. There were many difficult challenges early on. Among them was balancing the working groups' attention on health concerns that were of equal importance and of similar complexity, such as asthma. In addition, the immediate question was how to implement a strategy that would gain traction and have some early success, without losing sight of the need to tackle the more systemic policy problems (i.e., food availability and safe places for recreation) that would require a longer sustained commitment.

To get started we needed manpower. Fortunately, I was in a position to search for students seeking master's degrees in public health and interested in the topic of obesity and diabetes. I easily found Neetu Godwani, an intern, to get the program started. She quickly completed an assessment of the number of programs that were currently available in New York and in northern Manhattan that focused on nutrition and physical activity. The outcome of Godwani's assessment was neither surprising nor promising: northern Manhattan had a dearth of programs addressing poor nutrition and inactivity.

Next, we needed to shape the program. We were guided by three overarching goals. First, we sought to increase community knowledge of relevant nutrition and exercise/activity facts. Second, we aimed to create new resources by using bicultural educational tools, equipping agencies to provide education, and increasing access to facilities for maintaining a healthy lifestyle (places to exercise and participate in other recreational activities, such as dancing or group exercise). Our third goal was to inform policy and advocate for long-term macro changes to ensure sustainability of program goals, objectives, and activities. These were ambitious goals, and we decided to take them one step at a time.

Pilot Program at George Washington High School

We decided to start with a pilot program at a single site and selected George Washington High School for several reasons. Not only is it one of New York City's largest high schools and located in the heart of northern Manhattan, but also the school's leaders had expressed an clear interest in establishing a nutrition and wellness program. In addition, Walid Michelen, chair of the HP/DP working group, had already developed a great working relationship with the principal and assistant principal of the school. Finally, the age of the high school population addressed a concern of mine. I was convinced that too much attention was being focused on younger children, specifically those too young to make decisions on their own about what and where to eat. The Centers for Disease Control and Prevention, the New York State Department of Health, and others had begun to invest in programs aimed at younger children, but not enough attention was being placed on teens and young adults who were now faced with health problems, such as type II diabetes, that were unheard of in past generations. So, under the leadership of Walid Michelen and Sally Findley, the working group cochair, we embarked on a partnership with the school.

What the school wanted was a culturally relevant and interactive program that would engage parents, students, and staff and give them the tools to adopt healthy lifestyles. After multiple meetings with the school principal, assistant principals, teachers, and parents, it was clear to us that any initiative needed to increase motivation without stigmatization. Also, although diabetes and obesity were of great concern, the school leadership understood that it would be to the benefit of the parents and staff to capitalize the time dedicated to wellness courses and link them to other medically important topics, like high blood pressure, heart disease, and cancer. A more comprehensive and inclusive approach to the program would equip parents and staff to become health champions, not only for the families but also for the residents in the communities in which they lived and worked. This, of course, was very much in line with the Community Voices approach—it represented an opportunity to embed the community health worker training model into the school system and strengthen human capital in the Washington Heights and Harlem communities. Also, subcommittee members were convinced that good nutrition needed to be linked to overall wellness and health as well as to weight or body image. This required that we shift from the "diet" paradigm to the more encompassing "nutrition" and "healthy choices." Thus "Healthy Choices" was born, a program consisting of three components—a youth program, an adult program, and a written curriculum.

The Youth Program

We began by focusing on young adults. Youth are constantly bombarded with mixed messages in the media regarding body image and at the same time are marketing targets for America's leading fast-food chain restaurants. The challenge for us was twofold. First, how could we create a curriculum that would engage young adults as they emerge as the primary decision makers in food choices? Second—and more important—how could we channel their creativity and collective voice to speak up against the insidious marketing campaigns aimed at them from fast-food restaurants, soft drink companies, and calorie-empty food producers?

At the time, there were no formal nutrition curriculums in George Washington High School's health classes. In fact, the teachers and principals expressed serious concern that the health books provided by the Department of Education had not been updated since the 1980s. Thus, the "health teachers" (who actually where English and social studies teachers taking on the role of health teachers) felt ill equipped to teach and lead relevant discussions on health, nutrition, and wellness for these teenagers. What a missed opportunity! Here was a forty-minute time slot for young adults to sit in a required class, but they were not given the tools that would equip them to live healthy lives. What was more disturbing about the missed opportunity was that one of the schools within George Washington High School was a health professions specialty school (there are four schools with specific specialty areas). Students who had elected into this school within George Washington High School had a defined interest in entering the field of health and health care in college or in the workforce upon graduation. How could we not attend to this opportunity and invest time and other resources in supporting the schools effort in equipping these students to be health providers, experts, and leaders?

And so, in the summer of 2002, we took on the challenge. Healthy Choices, under the leadership of the Cornell-Cooperative Extension, one of the partnering organizations, and the support of Neetu Godwani, the MPH candidate I had selected as a Community Voices intern, designed a nutrition curriculum that would be integrated into George Washington's ninth- and eleventh-grade health classes. The curriculum had four main modules: Body Image, Nutrition 101, Relationship of Diet and Health Outcome, and Community Asset Mapping. Healthy Choices introduced the pilot curriculum in the spring 2003. We completed two consecutive semesters, and approximately thirty students participated in and successfully completed the course.

The Adult Program

Next, we turned our attention to interested adults. In this case, we already had something to build on. One of our youth program partners, the Cornell-Cooperative Extension, had an existing Eat Smart New York program tailored for adults and decision makers in the home environment. All we needed was to tweak the courses offered as a component of the Healthy Choices initiative to allow more of the Dominican-influenced cuisine to be part of the workshops on preparing healthier dishes. The Eat Smart New York program was uniquely flexible and would allow the content of the program to reflect the interest and cultural background of the primary audience: the parents of students and the staff members of George Washington High School. To this tested nutrition program we added exercise classes so the women learned how nutrition and exercise work together to build a healthy body.

The program was launched in the fall of 2003. The two-hour classes met Tuesdays, once a week, for eight weeks. The group of seventeen women met at the high school to learn how to live healthier by making informed choices about nutrition and exercise. Although it was open to all adults in the community, the participants were the mothers, aunts, and grandmothers of students attending the high school.

We held the classes at George Washington High School, where there were neither a state-of-the-art gym filled with treadmills and elliptical machines nor a fancy kitchen. Fortunately, this did not stop the women from participating. Classes were conducted in Spanish and started with an hour lesson on nutrition, moved into a half-hour hands-on cooking demonstration, and ended with thirty minutes of exercise. All the teaching, cooking, and exercising were done in the same classroom. A community educator from the Cornell-Cooperative Extension led the nutrition and cooking classes, and various guest instructors led the exercise and specialty workshops (for example, Diabetes 101, Cardiovascular Disease, and Health Insurance). For cooking lessons, the instructor brought an electric burner that plugged into the classroom's only electrical outlet. The women learned about the importance of including fresh fruits and vegetables in their diet. The class emphasized familiar fruits and vegetables—not just Western-centric vegetables such as spinach and broccoli—and drew from richer and more diverse categories like beets, papaya, and eggplants. Topics included, but were not limited to

- preparing and cooking quick, easy, low-cost meals
- sharing tips on food budgeting and menu planning
- learning about basic nutrition and how to read labels on food products
- stretching the food dollar while shopping

The majority of women were from the Dominican Republic and were motivated by a desire to help their families be healthier. In an article written for a departmental newsletter by Tamara Cannon, communications specialist of the Center for Community Partnerships, participants were quoted as saying, "I want to eat healthier, this way I can teach my children how to eat healthy" and "I decided to take these classes because of all the health issues in my family." Some mentioned specific information they learned; for example: "My family doesn't really notice when I use less oil, but I have noticed they have more energy. They have lost weight." Another explained the benefits this way: "There were many important things I never could understand, how to read the nutrition labels, the different food groups . . . carbohydrates, fibers, and minerals found in foods. Now I feel confident in what I have learned."

The half-hour physical activity highlighted movements to increase flexibility and endurance. Dersa Gonzalez, a parent coordinator at the school, and Yisel Alonzo, the Community Voices program coordinator, were in charge of this component. They tailored physical activity to the participants' interests. For example, they taught salsa dancing, which was an exciting and fun way to integrate flexibility and strength training with a culturally familiar activity. It was also an opportunity for the participants to socialize and connect as one community.

Almyra Ayos, the dance instructor, told Cannon, "By offering a dance class in salsa, the women not only learn the basic steps and rules, but can have fun. They also learn to make the connection between nutritional health and exercise, and motivate themselves—using music they enjoy— to move their bodies and to stay physically and mentally fit. Dance works wonders, not just for what it does to the body, but for what it does for the heart and mind." A participant agreed: "The salsa class is fun and interesting for me. As soon as I began to dance, I forgot about my stresses and go home energetic and tense-free." Another said, "You can't even imagine how much these classes have had an effect on my daily life. For example, before the course, and I'm embarrassed to share, I used to consume the same amount of calories you're supposed to eat in three days in one day. Now, I no longer eat that way. I eat healthier and not as much."

Upon completion of the ten-week adult course, we held a closing ceremony. For this occasion, the participants prepared potluck dishes of healthy recipes they learned in the class and were given a formal certificate of completion from Cornell University. Between 2003 and 2006 more than fifty women participated in the class, and forty received certificates of achievement.

Complements to the Healthy Choices Program

At the request of our partners, we also incorporated some additional components to complement the Healthy Choices program and use existing resources embedded in the institutions of our partners. Isabella, a geriatric center and one of the NMCVC Nutrition and Wellness partners, had already started a summer walking program for senior citizens called Walking Works Wonders. In an effort to enhance this program and partner with its neighbor George Washington High School, the center wanted to extend it to include youth from the school and open opportunities for parents to also participate. It worked! Youth and parents signed up to participate in this Saturday initiative, and Cornell-Cooperative Extension complemented the walking group with a nutrition workshop to reinforce the message of healthy eating and complete wellness. The nutrition workshop was offered immediately following the thirty-minute walks. In addition to the information that was shared, the workshops offered a venue for senior residents from Isabella, the youth from the community, and the students' parents to network and socialize. Although we did not evaluate this element of the program by interviewing participants, it was obvious from the energy of the room that the intergenerational connections were very special to all the participants. The Healthy Choices program was also complemented by a physician-led obesity support group at New York Presbyterian Hospitals Ambulatory Care Network to assist patients in their efforts to lose weight.

The Quest for Sustainability and Leadership

By 2006 Healthy Choices had two main components: the cooking and nutrition workshops that were offered to George Washington High School staff and parents, and the two-week curriculum in Nutrition and Wellness offered to eleventh and twelfth graders. We also had two linked, complementary components: the Walking Works Wonders program and the physician-led obesity groups.

The parent coordinators at George Washington High School, the principal and assistant principal, and the parents were extremely pleased with the content of the Healthy Choices program and were looking forward to continuing its existence. The parent coordinator made plans to increase outreach efforts in the community to promote the program. The participants and graduates of the class were able to share their experience with their peers, and as a result, there was always a group of interested parents waiting expectantly for the next series to begin. The Nutrition and Wellness Committee was delighted that the program took hold at the school and in the community. It gave us the early success we needed: a program was designed and successfully implemented. We had even gathered pre- and postsurvey data that showed that knowledge and behavior had been positively affected because of the program. Interviews with parents had confirmed the positive impact of the program.

But the troubling fact is that Healthy Choices was not fully sustainable. Although we did uncover a desire in parents and kids to become healthier, the conditions were not right for it to continue. As Yisel Alonzo observed,

"We simply didn't have the manpower or the funding to keep it going. We wished we did, but the reality was, it wasn't there."

This was a great disappointment to us since we both had worked hard and believed so passionately in the concept of the program, and the focus had been on young adults, family, and community. I (Jacqueline Martínez) had been a premed undergraduate at Cornell University but was not convinced that the basic practices of medicine would have any lasting impact on changing the health outcomes of individuals, let alone a community. In my opinion, prescribing medications to treat an illness might be effective, but the places people lived in, worked in, and played in had a more significant influence on their ability to recover and, in many cases, were an underlying cause of their current health conditions. My own experience with social and environmental disparities was what drove me to a career in public health in the first place. I was disappointed that so much of the emphasis in public health had turned to behavioral lifestyle choices at the individual level, especially in the early public health interventions addressing the HIV/AIDS epidemic. My training as a public health professional abroad and subsequently in Washington Heights at Columbia University Mailman School of Public Health gave me the tools and arsenal to tackle this new threat to the public's health from an environmental and social perspective. Like tobacco control, the obesity and diabetes crisis has given the public health field an opportunity to reclaim its historic role as a change agent focused on the environment and public policy. This initiative, Healthy Choices, was one way to express that thinking.

That having been said, when I look back at the project I am filled with an immense amount of pride and optimism. Despite the fizzled ending, this project was successful during its short life. When I ask myself, "What made this project succeed?" the answer becomes very clear—the leadership and dedication of two special women: Yisel Alonzo and Dersa Gonzalez. All the parent coordinators were advocates of the program, but Gonzalez stands out. She fought against unforeseen challenges (space, time, lack of financial resources) and pushed to insist that the program became a trademark of George Washington, securing its presence semester after semester for three years at the school. She and Alonzo were not only the champions of the program but also the change agents to impart a form of sustainability. Without them, the collective resource would not have taken hold in the community. And thanks to them, a group of people was empowered to take what they learned from the initiative and influence their neighbors, friends, and families to make health and wellness a priority in their lives. In the next section, Yisel Alonzo tells her story.

Sancocho (Yisel Alonzo)

When I joined the Community Voices initiative in 2003, I initially worked on the Health Information Tool for Empowerment project (see chapter 8). Although that project was exciting and satisfying, Healthy Choices struck a special chord in me. I am Dominican and had lived for many years in the heart of northern Manhattan, and the people who needed a program like Healthy choices were my people. My life, my reality, included direct experience with weight problems and diabetes. My uncles have diabetes. My grandfather died from it. My siblings are overweight and have high cholesterol, and I worry about getting diabetes myself. Weight has always been a struggle for me; my whole family has struggled with their weight. The reality of my life while growing up in that community at that time was this: we were afraid to go outside, afraid to play. For us, television became a safe haven of the inside, of being away from the danger and chaos of the outside, of street life. We did not even go to the park because of the gang activity and riots there. So, I understand firsthand how housing, education, and employment had the power to change the health of families and entire communities.

So, I did my best to pull together the individual components of the Healthy Choices initiative. I worked persistently to enhance the courses for parents, bringing in new and uncovered resources (such as salsa classes), and constantly communicating with the parents and parent coordinators to ensure the topics discussed were responsive to them and reflected their interest. I nurtured relationships with the parents and parent coordinators and tried to instill a sense of ownership of this initiative in them. I worked hard to make sure that the existence of this program also became a vehicle for community residents to feel welcomed, and that the program would be received as an opportunity to explore career changes and opportunities.

In the first year I was in the program, I began to understand how my voice, my efforts, and my talents could not only influence individual lives but also move existing structures to create and sustain something for the improvement of an entire community. I had long conversations with Jacqueline Martínez and others and began to explore the possibilities of furthering my education to maximize my skills and talents. After months of weighing my options, I decided to enroll into the master's in education program at Teachers College of Columbia University. Two years later I received my master's degree.

In the meantime, the NMCVC had decided to develop our own upgraded Healthy Choices curriculum. I worked on this component for about one year, along with Sara Timen, an MPH degree candidate at Columbia University who had a substantial background in teaching. The curriculum was based on what we had pulled together and learned from our pilot program— I think of it as a *sancocho*, a flavorful Dominican stew made from a little bit of everything. We had hoped this new curriculum would be the legacy that would be used to continue the program in George Washington High School and spread to other schools and community institutions. However, due to lack of funding, it was never piloted or even translated into Spanish. Today, it sits on a bookshelf, like a rich sancocho waiting to be served.

Room for Success

From 2003 to 2006 the Northern Manhattan Community Voices Collaborative Healthy Choices program was developed and implemented in one high school. Community efforts such as these are critical to reverse the trend of the obesity and diabetes epidemic. We know that Healthy Choices is a powerful tool that should, and could, be replicated among other communities throughout New York City. In fact, it is a program that the Department of Education should take up as its own and institute across schools in New York State. Although Healthy Choices was not sustainable, as is the case with the other NMCVC projects that met with only partial or short-lived success, there are lessons to be gleaned from the experience. The important lessons that were learned or reinforced as part of this program include:

- *Collaboration is essential.* Healthy Choices involved a hospital, a university, a local nutrition program, a local high school, and a senior and long-term care institution. To capitalize on an asset, a clear understanding of the existing resources is critical and has to be accompanied by a willingness to strengthen them and not re-create what others have done.

- *Input is a necessary ingredient.* A responsive program that reflects the immediate needs of a community requires input from the recipients of services every step of the way—from the design to the implementation to the evaluation of a project.
- *Champions help pave the way.* You need committed champions who understand the needs of a community and are willing to go the distance in insisting that it gets implemented. Yisel Alonzo and Dersa Gonzalez were two of the champions that did not allow institutional barriers get in the way of launching and maintaining a program.
- *Recognize your key components.* In our case, this was a committed leadership, a willingness to link and strengthen existing assets, and a school as the hub for implementation.

This chapter began with an emphasis on changing the underlying environmental forces that led to this unfortunate crisis in our nation. Programs like Healthy Choices are an important part of the equation. They create a vehicle to ignite local leadership and a method to address the immediate concern (knowledge and individual changes we can make in the midst of lack of other opportunities). But programs such as Healthy Choices are only part of the solution. Without the sustained commitment of institutions, government, private foundations, and community organizations to change the underlying policies that undermine individual choices, we will not see a palpable difference in the rates of obesity and diabetes threatening this country. Community organizations, parents, teachers, and other leaders need to be involved in a larger strategy: to inform policies that will hold accountable the corporations that have been targeting our youth and are unhealthy sources of food for our families; to demand equal access to safe playgrounds and areas for physical activity including affordable and accessible gym facilities; to push for changes in school policies that will reinstate the role of physical activity in the daily lives of youth and children; and to increase the availability of supermarkets that offer fresh and affordable produce in low-income neighborhoods. It is easy to tell people they need to eat healthy and exercise—actually most people already know this. The harder, but necessary, issue to face head-on is to address the underlying inequalities that hinder health and wellness in any community.

References

Berger, D. K., C. W. McCord, and T. R. Frieden (2003). Diabetes prevention and management. *City Health Information* 22, no. 3: 1–8.

Centers for Disease Control and Prevention (2009). *Childhood overweight and obesity.* http://www.cdc.gov/nccdphp/dnpa/obesity/childhood/.

—— (2003). *National diabetes fact sheet: U.S., 2003.* http://www.cdc.gov/diabetes/pubs/pdf/ndfs_2003.pdf.

—— (2007). *Health, United States, 2007.* Hyattsville, Md.: Centers for Disease Control and Prevention, National Center for Health Statistics.

—— (2009). *National Diabetes Surveillance System: Incidence of diabetes.* http://www.cdc.gov/diabetes/statistics/incidence_national.htm.

—— (2009). *Diabetes Surveillance System: Prevalence of diabetes.* http://www.cdc.gov/diabetes/statistics/prevalence_national.htm.

Frank, L., M. Andresen, and T. Schmid (2004). Obesity relationships with community design, physical activity, and time spent in cars. *American Journal of Preventive Medicine* 27, no. 2: 87–96.

Heath, G., et al. (2006). The effectiveness of urban design and land use and transport policies and practices to increase physical activity: A systematic review. *Journal of Physical Activity and Health* 3 (Suppl. 1): S55–76.

Kahn, E. B., et al. (2002). The effectiveness of interventions to increase physical activity: A systematic review. *American Journal of Preventative Medicine* 22, no. 4S: 73–107.

Knowler, W. C., et al. (2002). Reduction in the incidence of type 2 diabetes with lifestyle intervention or metformin. *New England Journal of Medicine* 346: 393–403.

Kriska, A. M, et al. (1986). A randomized exercise trial in older women: Increased activity over two years and the factors associated with compliance. *Medicine & Science in Sports & Exercise* 18: 557–62.

Leadership for Healthy Communities (2009). *Supporting Healthy Communities through the American Recovery and Reinvestment Act of 2009.* http://65.181.142.130/images/stories/lhc_policybrief_econ_4.6.09_final.pdf.

Linenger, J. M., C. V. Chesson, and D. S. Nice (1991). Physical fitness gains following simple environmental change. *American Journal of Preventative Medicine* 7: 298–310.

Lombard, D. N., T. N. Lombard, and R. A. Winett (1995). Walking to meet health guidelines: The effect of prompting frequency and prompt structure. *Health Psychology* 14: 164–70.

Mota, J., M. Almeida, P. Santos, and J. Ribeiro (2005). Perceived neighborhood environments and physical activity in adolescents. *Preventive Medicine* 41, nos. 5–6: 834–36.

Pratt, M., C. A. Macera, and C. Blanton (1999) Levels of physical activity and inactivity in children and adults in the U.S.: Current evidence and research issues. *Medicine & Science in Sports & Exercise* 31, no. 11S1: S526–33.

Reger, B., et al. (2002). Wheeling Walks: A community campaign using paid media to encourage walking among sedentary older adults. *Preventive Medicine* 35: 285–92.

Roux, L., et al. (2008). Cost effectiveness of community-based physical activity interventions. *American Journal of Preventive Medicine* 35, no. 6: 578–88.

Transportation Research Board and Committee on Physical Activity, Health, Transportation, and Land Use, Institute of Medicine of the National Academies (2005). *Does the built environment influence physical activity? Examining the evidence.*

U.S. Department of Health and Human Services (2003). *Prevention makes common "cents."* Washington, D.C.: U.S. Department of Health and Human Services.

Young, D. R., W. L. Haskell, C. B. Taylor, and S. P. Fortmann (1996). Effect of community health education on physical activity knowledge, attitudes, and behavior (the Stanford Five-City Project). *American Journal of Epidemiology* 144: 264–74.

Selected Additional References

Isabella website. http://www.isabella.org/.

Public Health Association of New York City (2007). *Reversing the diabetes and obesity epidemics in New York City: A call to action to confront a public health, economic and moral threat to New York City's future* (for a description of the obesity and diabetes epidemics in New York City).

Part IV

Providing Dental and
Mental Health Care

This part gives an account of how the Northern Manhattan Community Voices Collaborative addressed ways to improve the manner in which dental care is provided and the complex issues surrounding the provision of mental health care in the community. Insurance coverage for dental and mental health care often is left out, and as a result communities suffer from an inability to receive such care. The planning, development, and establishment of a new primary care medical and dental center in Harlem are described.

11

Columbia Community DentCare Program

STEPHEN MARSHALL, DAVID ALBERT, and DENNIS MITCHELL

Is the role of the dental school mainly to educate the next generation of dentists and create new knowledge? Or is there in addition a special need to consider the school's role in a community, especially when the community in which the school is located is in desperate need of care?

In the early 1990s several concurrent events laid the foundation for the Columbia Community DentCare Program. These events led to what we describe in this chapter as the "perfect storm." All of these influences were necessary to create this unique and remarkable program. Community Dent-Care consists of school-based dental centers, community practices, liaisons and partnerships with community-based organizations and faith-based groups, and linkages to public and private medical centers. Community DentCare began in the Washington Heights and Inwood communities of northern Manhattan and then broadened and expanded to include Harlem. This chapter tells the story of the development of the program and its maturation into the community service arm of the Columbia University College of Dental Medicine. We describe both how Community DentCare came about as well as its importance to the Community Voices initiative.

Underpinnings

During the early 1990s Columbia University's College of Dental Medicine, formerly known as the School of Dental and Oral Surgery, was going through major internal changes. These changes were the result of a strategic redirection of the school's missions and financial challenges. The former came about from a successful national grant project funded by the Pew Foundation urging dental schools to strengthen themselves to cope with ongoing changes in the profession and society; the latter was the result of withdrawal of New York State funding to support the enrollment of New York State students in private medical and dental schools. Because of these two catalysts in the early 1990s, College of Dental Medicine faculty and administration were accustomed to the idea that business as usual was not the case at the dental school. Generally, change in academic institutions and especially in professional schools is glacial at best. Every so often, however, great academic institutions recognize that the world around them has changed and that staying in synch requires a corresponding and swift transition on their part as well. Although the dental school at Columbia has always been well respected, the Pew grant and the financial challenges forced the faculty to realize that change was necessary to survive. Thanks to this established atmosphere of change, the idea and the reality of Community DentCare flourished within the university community and the school.

While change was afoot in the dental school in the early 1990s, it was mostly directed internally, toward the academic mission of teaching and research and the operation of the school's dental clinics. All dental schools operate dental clinics where the students gain experience in treating patients. These clinics are best described as "teaching" clinics because the main goal is education of students and not the efficient provision of care. However, the main goal for Community DentCare was conceived to be just the opposite: to provide efficient service in neighborhood locations outside of the walls of the dental school. Thus, Community DentCare was a dramatic departure from the usual academic mission of teaching and research. As a result, the school had to think about how best to treat an entire community and create a population-based delivery system. Academic institutions do not generally take responsibility for providing service at this level; in medical education, this is the role of the hospitals with which medical schools affiliate. Therefore, we had no model on which to pattern ourselves—in time, DentCare became a new role for dental schools.

In the early 1990s Washington Heights saw a rapid increase in population. The community has a history of immigration and accomplishment.

TABLE 11.1
Making a Difference: Community DentCare

PROBLEM

Northern Manhattan African American and Latino children have worse disease
  than others
Dental caries in all adolescents: United States: 17%; northern Manhattan: 37%
Dental caries in African Americans: United States: 31%; northern Manhattan:
  50%
Dental caries in Latinos: United States: 27 %; northern Manhattan: 33%
Dental caries in whites: United States: 13%
Teeth that need extraction or root canal: All: 8%; African Americans: 18%;
  Latinos: 6%

SOLUTION

Community DentCare, a new model that integrates community dental care in a
  teaching school

RESULTS

School prevention sites: 11,000 visits per year
Mobile van: 3,000 visits per year
Neighborhood practices: 30,000 visits per year

Note: Percentages have been rounded up or down.

Source: Mitchell (2003).

Waves of immigrants have populated the area, with first and second generations moving out to other areas of New York and the United States. One
hundred years ago German immigrants moved to the area from the squalid
tenements of the Lower East Side of New York City. Former secretary of
state Henry Kissinger is a notable immigrant to the area. He was the child
of immigrants who settled in the area and then moved on, embodying the
American dream. In addition to German immigrants, large groups of Irish,
Jewish, and Italian immigrants made Washington Heights/Inwood (WH/I)
their home. Following these groups came Puerto Ricans in the 1960s and
1970s. Immigrants from the Dominican Republic supplanted them, with
substantial growth in the Dominican population occurring in the 1990s.
In recent years immigrants from Central America have settled into the
community. It was within this dynamic "melting pot" that Community
DentCare found its roots.

To understand the birth of Community DentCare, it is important to understand the community's unique geography as well. Although they are inhabitants of a large metropolitan area, the residents of WH/I live within a geographically isolated community. The island of Manhattan is 12 miles long from north to south and only 2.5 miles wide at its widest point. In northern Manhattan it narrows to only a few blocks in width. This is the area known as Washington Heights/Inwood. It is bounded on the west by the Hudson River, on the east and north by the Harlem River, and to the south by 155th Street. There are several small bridges that link the community to the West Bronx on the east and north sides. The George Washington Bridge provides a connection to New Jersey to the west. The communities to the east in the Bronx have chronic poverty and poor medical and dental services. To access New Jersey and its more affluent suburban communities requires a costly bus ride or paying a toll and traveling via car. To the south of WH/I is Harlem, a community with chronic poverty that has been designated a Health Manpower Shortage Area by the Health Resources and Services Bureau of Health Professions. In the early 1990s the official New York City census listed for Harlem a population of approximately 150,000 inhabitants; however, it was generally agreed that the population exceeded 200,000 when undocumented aliens were taken into account.

"Our Children Have Toothaches"

The story begins with a letter that then dean Allan Formicola received from Phyllis Williams, the principal of one of the local public schools in Washington Heights. Her letter was a plea for help. She explained that she had children with toothaches sitting outside her office with no place to send them for treatment. She said this was a common occurrence, and she was turning to the dean of the dental school for a solution. The dean responded that he would think about the problem and try to find a grand solution, but in the meantime she could send the children to our teaching clinic for treatment. At the time he realized that his response was only a bandage on the bigger problem; that most of the children in all the schools in northern Manhattan were not getting preventive dental care, and few had access to regular treatment. Yes, the school's teaching clinics treated children, but usually by the time those children came in they were suffering from advanced dental disease. In fact, each year Columbia pediatric dentists needed to bring over one hundred young children to the operating room to treat severe conditions as a result of neglected dental disease. Most people do not like to go to the dentist, and in underserved communities where children have little to no access to dentists they find their way to the school's clinics only when in pain. Furthermore, our dental school clinics are in the midst of the Columbia University Medical Center and can be very difficult to locate.

The dean brought together the three of us as we were each trained in public health and in dentistry. He challenged us: Could there be a different more active approach for the dental school to pursue, one in which we could reach out into the community to prevent disease and treat it earlier? Is the role of the dental school mainly to educate the next generation of dentists and create new knowledge? Or is there in addition a special need to consider the school's role in a community, especially when the community in which the school is located is in desperate need of care? These were the weighty questions that the principal's letter stimulated within our dental school.

The responsibility for thinking about such questions and then setting the direction for initiatives that may result from them usually falls on the dean's shoulders. However, as Henry Rosovsky, former dean of the Faculty of Arts and Sciences at Harvard University, points out, deans are tightly scheduled all day long, meeting with faculty, alumni, and administrators, with little to no uninterrupted time to "write, read, think, or dream." But in developing a plan to deal with the community dental problems, that is exactly what it takes: time to think carefully about the problem, time to write a clear plan around a bold vision or dream. The dean developed a team effort to think through and plan the effort. We became the leaders in that effort.

By 1992 the dental school had come through the major internal changes directed by its strategic plan and had recovered from its financial challenges. A dedicated group of faculty, many of whom were recently appointed to assist the senior faculty, worked on implementing the internal changes to the educational programs and improving the efficiency of the operation of the large teaching clinics. With this forward movement as a backdrop, the dean began to discuss Principal Williams's letter with the faculty as well as the larger issue of determining the school's role in interacting with the community to put into place preventive care and early treatment. He was convinced that something needed to be done. The data from the teaching clinics at Columbia indicated that we were treating mainly very young children with very severe disease, and that adolescents and teenagers were not seeking care. In addition, we were experiencing an influx of young adults in their twenties with severe disease, a sure sign that the community was lacking a preventive approach to oral disease.

The Wheel-Spokes-Hub Approach

Each of us took on different roles in developing the Community DentCare program. First, one of us (David Albert) looked at the manpower in northern Manhattan to see if there was a sufficient workforce for the population. Albert and his staff conducted a street-by-street, office-by-office assessment of the current dental resources in the community. It became apparent that the community lacked adequate access to dental care. The federal government concurred, and it designated the community as a dental Manpower Shortage Area. This designation remains today for both WH/I and Harlem. The assessment leading up to the dental manpower shortage application revealed how few dental services were present. Outside of the Columbia University College of Dental Medicine clinics, there were virtually no specialty services. Only one part-time oral surgeon practiced, on 181st Street. One orthodontist was present in Washington Heights and one in Inwood. The oral surgeon and orthodontists were located within middle-class pockets in the community. In making this application we also found that the two most impoverished census tracts in New York City were located in WH/I. Albert began to discuss with WH/I community leaders priorities for an intervention. Dennis Mitchell took on the assignment to discuss priorities with Harlem community leaders. The administration of a community effort fell under the purview of the assistant dean, Stephen Marshall, hired to implement the strategic changes in the mid-1980s, who worked closely with the dean.

In response, we began to sketch out the overall blueprint of Community DentCare. Albert described it as a wheel-spokes-hub approach where the prevention programs in the public schools were the spokes and the treatment centers the hub of the wheel. All realized that setting up prevention clinics in the public schools was a good approach; however, children with dental disease, mainly dental caries, would also require treatment. The plan would need to make sure that treatment could happen in spite of the fact that there were not sufficient numbers of willing practitioners in the community to treat the children. So in addition to the prevention sites, it was necessary to set up community-based clinics and lists of referral private practices that would be willing to treat the children.

The plan was shaping up, and we were getting more and more excited; however, we ran into a speed bump in Harlem. The Harlem planning group, headed by Mitchell, learned that in addition to the focus on children there was a significant need to provide care for older people, who had also long been neglected. This bump in the road led to its own solution: the development of the Thelma C. Davidson Adair Medical/Dental Center in Harlem (see chapter 13).

Marshall superimposed the wheel-spokes-hub plan on a large map of northern Manhattan. We all felt inspired by the grand design, the dream. There are twenty-eight schools in northern Manhattan, and the plan envisioned eventually reaching children in all of them. National data indicated that dental disease levels in racial and ethnic minority groups were considerably higher than in whites. Various studies conducted by the dental school for the New York State Department of Health indicated that the incidence of caries in African American and Latino children was high. Since northern Manhattan was largely an African American and Latino community, we were sure that from those studies carried out by the faculty and from the reports from the school principals, we would be seeing children with severe disease once the program was implemented.

Presenting the Community DentCare Plan

At a regular administrative meeting of the health science schools leadership, the dean described the dental needs of northern Manhattan and, using Marshall's map, presented the solution—the Community DentCare plan. Since the problems and issues discussed at these meetings led by the vice president of health sciences were usually internal, the community plan piqued their interest. The dean was pleasantly surprised at the encouraging reception the plan received from the medical center leadership.

Next, the dean and Marshall presented the plan to a group at the State Health Department. Their response was a different story. Instead of encouraging us, one of the officials who dealt with Medicaid accused us of designing a plan solely to "make money for the dental school" from Medicaid funding. We were completely floored, and the dean angrily took great exception to his charge, pointing out that many of the children had no Medicaid coverage and that we would treat all children regardless of the ability to pay. The dean pointed out that this was not a plan from a fly-by-night for-profit group, but one coming from a nonprofit academic institution with high ethical standards. We were not convincing enough and the meeting ended with state officials believing the school would not find the resources to implement Community DentCare. Of course, this only heightened our desire to see the plan implemented.

Kellogg Comes Onboard

Fortunately, we had some resources to turn to in designing the implementation of the plan. In the 1980s the Columbia University School of Public Health (now the Joseph L. Mailman School of Public Health) had developed a school-based health clinic program that was in place in several intermediate schools. The leader of that program, Lorraine Tiezzi, and the dean of the School of Public Health were receptive to having us utilize the administrative infrastructure they had established in the schools to implement the dental preventive program. In addition, Columbia Presbyterian Hospital (now New York Presbyterian Hospital) ran off-site ambulatory clinics in which two dental clinics staffed by College of Dental Medicine faculty were already in place in northern Manhattan and another was under construction. The start of the wheel-and-hub model was a reality. But the development of the plan required more than that. It required startup funding, and for this the dean turned to the W. K. Kellogg Foundation.

At first, the foundation was reluctant to get involved and turned down appeals for a grant. However, the dean read between the lines of their turn-down letter and saw some hope. He persisted, and the Foundation agreed to send two of its project officers for a site visit. One of the site visitors was a dentist and the other a senior program officer. They requested not only to meet with faculty who had worked on developing the plan, but to meet with community representatives. In preparing for the latter, the dean met with Moisés Pérez, executive director of Alianza Dominicana. Pérez had met with Albert during the development of the plan, and the community affairs officer for the Health Science Schools, Ivy Fairchild, had discussed the plan with him. Now, in preparation for the Kellogg Foundation site visit, he was to meet with the dean face-to-face for the first time. Pérez was frankly wary of our motivation for the plan, since historically the prime motivation for university faculty's interest in the community was in doing research that had benefits for the school but little to no direct benefit for the community. The dean convinced Pérez that our plan put service first as its motivation and children's health up front. Pérez understood that the dental school would need to cover its costs and that research could come from implementing the plan; however, he was satisfied that our motivation for the plan stemmed from a sense of responsibility that the dental school was part of the community and as such needed to use its intellectual resources to better the community. This relationship with Pérez and Alianza Dominicana carried over into other cooperative efforts developed in the years that followed.

The site visit went well. The Kellogg Foundation's program officers recommended to the foundation that a grant of $1 million be awarded to launch Community DentCare. In a memorable moment, everyone who worked on the development of the plan signed a Kellogg's cereal box to celebrate the successful grant application and presented it the dean. The box still hangs in his office.

Now came the time to operationalize the plan. This was about the time that an imposing figure walked into Albert's community-based hospital practice. The practice was located across the street from Intermediate School (IS) 52. The gentleman identified himself as Leonard Latronica, the principal of IS 52. He indicated that he had heard about our work and wanted to know when we would start providing services at IS 52. He was a remarkably busy individual but had found the time to come to speak to Albert without calling or making an appointment. He indicated that when he was a child growing up in New York City there were few resources except a clinic that serviced children in need on the Upper East Side. He would visit that clinic and receive his care. He wanted to know why that was not the case here in WH/I and why we could not provide services at his school. He explained that his school was severely overcrowded, with 1,800 students in a building built for 1,200. Bathrooms had been converted to classrooms, yet he wanted to and was willing to take vital educational space and allocate it for a dental program. Albert asked him why, and his response was that on a daily basis he had children in dental pain in his office. He usually could not find a place to send these children for care, and he was offering us his help and assistance. Albert met with Latronica on a regular basis in his office at IS 52, where it became apparent that not only was he a principal and an educator, he was also a social worker, policeman, and planner. His insistence on a dental program was the catalyst that led to the first Community DentCare site.

The second school in which we put a preventive clinic in place was IS 143 in Washington Heights, the same school from which the original letter from the principal was written. Principal Williams was a big supporter of making sure children in her school had adequate access to health care. The existing health clinic operated by the School of Public Health helped provide the infrastructure, such as parental approvals to treat the children. The principal provided space for a small clinic in which a dental hygienist was assigned to provide preventive care. After the program began, Principal Williams was so happy with it that she assigned additional space so that a full dental practice with two treatment rooms could be built in order to allow a dentist to treat the children who needed care. Soon the clinic was very busy.

This success was repeated in several other schools in Washington Heights/Inwood and Harlem. Although the plan to have dental prevention programs in twenty-eight schools has not been realized, there are now seven school programs throughout northern Manhattan (IS 143, IS 52, IS 164, PS 180, IS 136, Thurgood Marshall Academy, and Promise Academy). The first spokes on the wheel were in place. (The hubs, the neighborhood community practices and the private practices to which children requiring treatment were to be referred, still needed to be developed.) In three of the schools (IS 143, IS 52, IS 164), full dental facilities were ultimately built so that the children could receive not only preventive treatment but also restorative care as well. The enthusiastic response from the principals helped to reward those faculty directly involved.

The Dental Van

Before discussing the development of the hubs, it is necessary to mention the mobile van. We realized that we wanted to get children into preventive care at an earlier age than we were able to do by focusing on children enrolled in intermediate public schools, where they were already 11 or 12 years old. One way to do this was to start a preventive program for Head Start children—another and different spoke in the wheel. We decided the best approach would be to use a mobile van that could move from one Head Start program to another.

Once again, finding funds to implement this project became a stumbling block—but not for long. One of us (Mitchell) convinced the Paula Vial Lempert Foundation to award a grant of $150,000 for the van. Then we developed a partnership with the Children's Aid Society as they also sought to improve the oral health of our community. The society already operated a van, but their van was old and needed to be replaced. So, we pooled resources and purchased a new, well-equipped van, 36 feet long with a 60-gallon gas tank. With such a behemoth, logistical issues surfaced right away: Where do you park a 36-foot van in Manhattan? We searched out one location after another. Finally, the director of athletics at the university gave us permission to park the van at Baker Field, the university's athletic field in upper Manhattan—with the proviso that we move the van when Columbia played its home football games. It is amazing now to reflect back and realize how big this parking problem was at the time and how much energy we all put into solving it. However, the van was the means to reach the Head Start children. Today, it is booked up five days a week and is in great demand. It received an annual grant from Proctor and Gamble for five years to assist in paying operational costs. The van is an important part of Community DentCare as it targets a vulnerable group where good oral health habits can be taught to both children and their parents. In fact, the original van was replaced in the fall of 2009 because it was so heavily used that we wore it out! And, we were delighted that the van program got the attention of Alex Rodriguez of the New York Yankees. His foundation made a $250,000 commitment for the new van and the work that it does in the community. A-Rod was there at the ceremony to cut the ribbon on the new van.

Creating the Hub

Now, back to the hub part of Community DentCare. The Harlem Hospital Dental Service and the dental school's main clinics in Washington Heights served as the referral site for complex treatment. Presbyterian Hospital did not follow through on its original commitment to include a dental facility in each of its off-site facilities. Instead, it permitted only one of its twenty-one ambulatory sites to include dental services, and this location focused on older people. That meant that we had to switch into search mode again and find other sites (and, in two cases, build them).

We located several existing dental programs in community health clinics that realized the benefits of affiliating with the dental school. We developed formal affiliation agreements with three community health centers over the years. In addition, the university built two new facilities (Thelma C. Davidson Adair Medical/Dental Center and Columbia University Haven Pediatric Practice). These health clinics were strategically located throughout the community and became referral sites for the Community DentCare network. In addition, Marshall found that the private practice dentists in Washington Heights wanted to participate in the plan. Working with leaders in the Dominican Dental Society, we worked out a plan with the assistance of Ivy Fairchild to include them as referral sites.

Our network was now in place, and residents and students from the dental school rotate to these sites to gain experience learning about the problems of the underserved. The educational experiences they gain open their eyes to the needs of the underserved. This is an important part of their education and training, and the DentCare plan therefore provides benefits beyond the 44,000 patient visits each year. If the health care system in the United States is to serve all of the people, then those in training must become understanding of the problems of those who are less fortunate in society.

Improving Access

Creating a broad, community-wide approach to improve access to dental care in an underserved community is an enormous undertaking, as national data indicate that the amount of care needed would be quite high due to the level of oral disease found in low-income communities. Mitchell carried out a study of the disease levels in the school children in northern Manhattan to compare them with the rest of the nation. The study showed that children in northern Manhattan had much higher disease levels and much less treated disease than those in the rest of the country. In fact, there are twice as many children with emergency situations than in the rest of the nation. The results of the study made us realize the enormity of the problem we had taken on.

Community DentCare was initiated in 1996, and by 2000 the surgeon general's first ever report on the oral health of Americans was published. The report outlined the need to deal with what was called a "silent" epidemic of oral disease and in particular pointed out the need in low-income communities where access to care was limited. During the rollout of the surgeon general's report, the dean made a presentation describing Community DentCare. Sitting in the audience was a program officer from the Robert Wood Johnson Foundation. After the presentation she came to visit us at Columbia and asked if we would help the foundation structure a national program to improve access to care. What resulted from that meeting was the largest foundation initiative on dentistry ever undertaken in the United States. Thanks to the Robert Wood Johnson Foundation and the joint involvement of two other foundations, W. K. Kellogg Foundation and the California Endowment, $26.3 million was invested in stimulating dental schools around the nation to become involved in the access to care issue. Columbia became the national program office for this huge initiative. Who would have dreamed that the letter from Principal Williams so many years ago would have led to this grand outcome? In another turn of events, the New York State Department of Health recently provided Community Dent-Care with a $1 million grant to build a comprehensive treatment clinic at IS 164 and replace our mobile van, which has reached the end of its useful life. The opening ceremony for the new clinic at I.S. 164 was held in May 2009 and the new van arrived in July 2009.

The Robert Wood Johnson Foundation project, "Pipeline, Profession & Practice: Community-Based Dental Education," funded fifteen dental schools in its first phase (2002–2007) to work on improving the knowledge, skills, and attitudes of the future practitioners to deal with access issues by connecting students to communities in their final year of dental school. An additional eight schools are being funded in the second phase (2008–2010), so that by the time the national program is concluded twenty-three dental schools, almost half of the schools in the nation, will have put their energies into this problem.

On a more local level, the philosophy behind Community DentCare has carried over into the development of the Northern Manhattan Community Voices Collaborative. Central to the underlying Community DentCare philosophy is that academic institutions must collaborate with their communities and must deal with the real problems they face. In so doing, everyone benefits. The community receives the knowledge and skills of the faculty in solving problems, and students gain experience by service learning from community residents. Most community leaders realize that in return, the community needs to assist the faculty in carrying out research, but they do not want to be just a means to the next research project. By collaborating, the community and the university meet on an equal playing field where all issues are put on the table and together solutions are found. While this founding principle of Community DentCare sounds like a simple philosophy, it is by no means easy to implement and to live by. There are many twists and turns for both parties. In the end, however, both community and academic institutions thrive when adhering to this philosophy.

References

Albert, D., et al. (2002). Dental caries among disadvantaged 3–4-year-old children in northern Manhattan. *Pediatric Dentistry* 24, no. 3: 229–33.

Foner, N. (2009). *Immigrant New York at the turn of the 21st century.* http://www
.africanart.org/uploads/resources/docs/nancy_foner_immigrants_sympo
sium_paper_5.26.09.pdf.

Formicola, A., et al. (1999). Population-based primary care and dental education: A new role for dental schools. *Journal of Dental Education* 63, no. 4: 331–38.

Mitchell, D., et al. (2003). Dental caries experience in northern Manhattan adolescents. *Journal of Public Health Dentistry* 63, no. 3: 189–204.

New York City Department of City Planning (2004). *The newest New Yorkers 2000.* http://www.nyc.gov/html/dcp/html/census/nny.shtml.

Perry, M. J., and P. J. Mackun (2000). *Population change and distribution 1990 to 2000.* Census 2000 Brief.

Rosovsky, H. (1990). *The university: An owner's manual.* New York: Norton.

U.S. Department of Health and Human Services (2000). *Oral health in America: A report of the surgeon general.* http://www.surgeongeneral.gov/library/oralhealth/.

12

Mental Health Policy Paper

Giving Voice to a Neglected Epidemic

LOURDES HERNÁNDEZ-CORDERO

The NMCVC created an action document for northern Manhattan providers and consumers of mental health services, whose recommendations served to guide the work of local community leaders, institutions, and traditional and nontraditional mental health service providers for years to come.

The story of the policy paper *Mental Health: The Neglected Epidemic* is a bit like the story of the ugly duckling: it seemed an odd bird from the moment it was hatched: it was a paper, not a program, and one whose potential was not universally recognized. But in the end, it grew into a useful document that, while perhaps not quite as beautiful as a swan, became something that people from many walks of life could rally around, appreciate, and use in their work.

The paper emerged from the Difficult to Cover Services working group, whose mandate was to conduct assessments and make recommendations about the delivery of mental and oral health services in northern Manhattan. The running joke among the collaboration partners was that the "dental/mental" working group dealt with both of these issues because they were located in the head. The proper explanation for putting these two issues together is how, historically, insurance coverage for both types of services is typically carved out of health insurance coverage. That is, dental coverage is usually separate from medical coverage and mental health services are often outsourced or cut, or when included they are limited in a different way from medical services. The Northern Manhattan Community Voices Collaborative leadership had a head start on the oral health side since one of the founding members of the collaborative included the Columbia School of Dental and Oral Surgery, and with them came a set of initiatives that were waiting to see the light of day (see chapters 11 and 13).

For mental health, though, the story was different. While the other two core collaboration partners—Alianza Dominicana and Harlem Hospital—had mental health programs, that was not their main area of work. Thus, to get an idea of where to go next, a policy paper seemed like the place to start. We instinctively knew that we would need to engage in a complex process of digging below the surface to stimulate deep changes with far-reaching effects. Subsequent research supported this approach but also stirred up considerable resistance that we needed to overcome. This chapter is the story of how the Difficult to Cover Services working group did just that, or how the ugly duckling turned into an action document for northern Manhattan providers and consumers of mental health services, whose recommendations served to guide the work of local community leaders, institutions, and traditional and nontraditional mental health service providers for years to come.

Forming the Committee

The first step in forming the committee was to convene the NMCVC partners involved in the provision of mental health services. The Community Voices team sought help from the Northern Manhattan Mental Health Council's cochair, Charles Corliss. Corliss is executive director of Inwood Community Services, which runs a mental health clinic and an outpatient addiction program. I teamed up with a research assistant and together we interviewed many researchers from the New York State Psychiatric Institute, but it was Roberto Lewis-Fernandez who took on an active role in the committee. Columbia University Medical Center's faculty Jennifer Haven and Mary McCord brought to the group their important insights on the special needs of children, while David Weng brought us up to speed on the education of new mental health professionals. To get an idea of the special needs of seniors, we reached out to the Washington Heights Inwood Coalition on Aging's Fern Hertzberg and the late Leslie Foster. In addition, we consulted other community-based practitioners such as Alianza Dominicana's Family Center, Upper Manhattan Mental Health Clinic, and Heritage Health and Housing (these last two groups are located in Harlem).

Consumers from various sites and family representatives linked with the National Alliance on Mental Illness were also engaged.

How I became involved in the committee is a story in itself, a story in which pure chance plays a central role. As a graduate student at the time, I had previously been working on a research project related to mental health. For that project I helped recruit patients and their families. This entailed visiting psychiatric emergency rooms and patient units in four local hospitals, identifying individuals who had been recently diagnosed with a mental illness with psychotic features and—if they were interested in participating—obtaining their informed consent to take part in the study. I then interviewed relatives identified by study participants to corroborate some of the information participants provided us. This part was the hardest. Over and over, relatives of the people experiencing their first psychotic break were struggling with making sense of their loved one's diagnosis, some of them asking themselves, "What did I do to cause this?" On the one hand, I was humbled by their openness. On the other hand, I was frustrated and feeling useless. Many of the experiences the interviewees and study participants shared with me did not fit into the interview form I was asked to fill out. Lacking the long-term experience and perspective necessary when conducting basic research, I struggled to see how what I was doing could help anyone.

This was not what I expected of public health, and for a moment I considered dropping the doctorate program in public health for one in health education. I had already applied to and was accepted by Teachers College when, by a stroke of luck, another door opened. The hands on the doorknob were the then head of the Sociomedical Sciences Department, Cheryl Healton, and my mentor Ana Abraido-Lanza. They both learned of my plans to switch doctorate programs. The department had recently lost two other Latina students, and losing a third one would not be an option. I met with them and shared the reasons for my unhappiness with the program— coursework that seemed too theoretical, not enough opportunities for practical applications or sharpening of professional skills. After all, I had chosen a DrPH over a PhD because I wanted a practical degree instead of an academic one. They understood my frustration and proposed that I consider the newly established Community Scholars program as part of the NMCVC.1 I was interviewed and accepted as a Community Scholar, and that decision shaped the rest of my career. As a Community Scholar, I was assigned to carry out the program coordination responsibilities for the

Difficult to Cover Services working group—specifically doing the research and writing the policy paper. I was charged with the task of compiling the data, juggling the schedules of overly stretched individuals, and balancing sometimes competing interests.

First Steps: Getting to Know the Lay of the Land

To produce the paper, the committee felt we first needed to learn about the status of mental health services in northern Manhattan. We also felt strongly that the paper should include the multiple perspectives of institutional and community-based practitioners, consumers, and the general public. We wanted an in-depth look at how community residents experienced mental health and illness on a day-to-day basis, the challenges faced by providers in their efforts to deliver culturally relevant quality care, and the view nonconsumers had of people living with mental illness. However, the skeptics—among them people who had been working in the field of mental health for a long time—told us that all that was needed to solve most of the problems was additional funding to support existing programs and increase the delivery of behavioral health services. It would have been easy to simply report that and work with the group in advocating for increased funding. In doing the initial research, however, I soon found out that filling the gaps in northern Manhattan's mental health landscape was a bit more complicated. So, even before beginning the task of producing a policy paper, we had to first convince some of the key stakeholders that it was worth their time to be part of the process to outline the situation and to analyze and set goals at multiple levels.

As I set out to learn about mental health services in northern Manhattan, certain national trends served to organize my search, since they were all reflected at the local level. National efforts to raise awareness around mental health issues were increasing, and in 1999 the White House Conference on Mental Health called for a national antistigma campaign while the surgeon general issued a *Call to Action on Suicide Prevention*. Shortly thereafter, these were followed by the surgeon general's report on mental health and a major national conference on Children's Mental Health. It was becoming clear that great advances in understanding mental illness, growing knowledge in the science of the brain, and the development of nonpharmaceutical therapeutic options unfortunately were not resulting in better mental health for Americans. In addition, disparities in access to mental health care were even wider than in other areas of health and medicine. In the general population, stigmatization and fear restrained millions of people from seeking help. Those who did take that first step faced a shortage of services. In addition, financial barriers and lack of parity in insurance coverage continued to be major obstacles to access.

Against this backdrop, and with the working group convened, I set out to document the state of mental health in northern Manhattan using a variety of methods. I conducted a series of interviews with key informants from community-based agencies and health care institutions serving children, adolescents, adults, and older people—with the first of these interviewees being the working group members themselves. As additional tasks were outlined, I was joined by Paola Mejía, who was also a graduate student and Community Scholar. Paola and I conducted a series of discussion groups with both consumers and nonconsumers of mental health services on sites that were either a part of Community Voices partner agencies or received services from them. We also conducted an inventory of organizations providing mental health care services. The inventory included questions on types of services, target population, number of clients served, yearly visits, waiting period, staff, and language capability. Finally, we analyzed citywide public data in order to obtain points of comparison with other neighborhoods. Paola and I talked with young people and older people, parents of school-aged children, men and women. For weeks, we barely set foot in our office! Tape recorder in hand and bearing gifts of snacks and refreshments, we covered key sites in northern Manhattan.

While Paola Mejía and I did most of the footwork, working group members were instrumental in reading drafts, writing sections, and making introductions that allowed Paola and me to gain entry into organizations that we had no previous relationships with. These introductions were worth their weight in gold—in public health, it is all about relationships.

Redefining Mental Health

Each resource made a unique contribution to our growing knowledge. Conversations with people who were not engaged in the mental health care system—nonconsumers, other health professionals—were particularly informative in so many ways. Perhaps the most important outcome from our group discussions was the insight that mental health is perceived as related to all spheres of daily life, not solely as illness, a medical or psychiatric problem to be treated with medication. In fact, mental health problems were largely attributed to stress derived from social, economic, and personal situations faced in daily life. These were mainly structural in nature: lack of affordable housing and the feeling of being pushed out of the neighborhood, poverty, violence, drugs, and unemployment surfaced in every discussion on mental health.

In an interview for this book, a community member told us about her daughter, who was the victim of sexual violence. "There was a man that tried to sexually abuse her and we ended up going to Alianza. They helped me with all the paperwork . . . gave me phone numbers of people that I could call . . . psychologists . . . that was an experience that made me feel that I was not alone."

Another community member points out that many people in northern Manhattan need "a lot of therapy." What kind? "Mental therapy," she said. "There are people that are suffering from domestic violence. A lot of young people don't know what they want out of life. It's difficult, but we have to help them. . . . A lot of young people have dropped out of school, they feel alone, some of their parents are drug addicts" (box 12.1).

BOX 12.1

Of Craziness and Illness

Here is what discussion group participants had to say when asked to describe *a person with mental illness*:

1. There is a difference between mental illness one was *born with* vs. being *a result of* one's own actions.
2. Mental illness that occurred in the elderly was perceived as *natural*, and something that comes *with age*.
3. Certain diagnoses were perceived as *character flaws*.

Most people giving these descriptions did not know any mentally ill people personally. Their opinion, participants admitted, was based on images of the mentally ill portrayed in the media.

With this broad view of mental health, Paola and I found that multiservice agencies that were working on initiatives oriented to alleviate individual burdens considered these efforts as indirect interventions to enhance mental health. Support services in housing, child care, training, employment, and community empowerment were proposed as effective prevention strategies. Given the characteristics of our community, services for newly arrived immigrants, regardless of their legal status, were felt as a poignant necessity.

Identifying Four Major Challenges

My conversations with mental health service providers were equally enlightening. I realized that the little bit of what I had learned about mental health was framed within the health care system; it was somewhat theoretical, and very little was based on firsthand experience. And there was the issue of money. At the time, members of the council feared the potential negative effect of the transition of Medicaid into managed care. We now know that it has indeed had a dramatic effect on service delivery for Medicaid clients. For example, Medicaid managed care has set limits on the number of treatment sessions per year, dramatically reduced hospital stays, and transferred most detoxification clients to outpatient settings. Although funding was an issue, slowly I came to the realization that the quick "we just need more money" assessment was not complete. Many of these challenges were not solely dependent on funding.

I learned that service providers confronted challenges in delivering quality care, mainly related to (1) the way funds and resources were allocated; (2) the limited capacity of the system to meet the existing need for services, especially for vulnerable populations; (3) the need for more personnel; and (4) the difference in priorities between providers and consumers.

The first challenge of allocating resources stemmed from the need to choose between treatment and prevention. I remember how over and over Moisés Pérez of Alianza Dominicana would point at the rocking chairs in the waiting area of the Family Center and the ladies huddled around them crocheting. To him, this opportunity to socialize and be neighborly was as valuable a piece of prevention as a social worker–run support group. Advocates for clinical treatment and advocates for preventive services were both aware of the devastating effects that living conditions in our community had on mental health (i.e., immigration status, uprooting, acculturation, substance abuse) and recognized the role that both prevention and treatment played in the delivery of services. Yet, at the existing funding level, it was hard to reconcile the dilemma between these two priorities. Try requesting support for creating spaces for crocheting! In the past, this dilemma had been addressed by targeting funding for paraprofessional staff to provide prevention and consultation services. The drawback, however, was that when these paraprofessionals were faced with diagnoses that were out of the scope of their training, they were forced to refer patients to agencies that had a waiting list or to send them to the psychiatric emergency room.

The second challenge was the problem of capacity to provide slots for consumers and effective follow-up. Both consumers and clinicians agreed that continuity of care was important, with continuity defined not only as having uninterrupted treatment, but also as being able to see the same provider over time. Debra Wilson, one of the consumers actively involved in the Northern Manhattan Mental Health Council, shared with me during a bus ride together that the problem with not being able to see the same provider consistently was that "you need to keep telling your story all over again" because seeing a clinician is much more than simply getting your medication adjusted on a regular basis. It is about having a trusting relationship with someone who knows "your story." These two conditions were difficult to maintain in a system with limited capacity. The problem with system capacity was seen as especially harsh to vulnerable populations: children, adolescents, older people, chronically mentally ill people, and immigrants.

The third challenge was filling the need for an array of personnel, including paraprofessionals, social workers, psychologists, and psychiatrists. For example, at the hospital level, one of the deterrents to having mental health professionals at the clinics was the complicated reimbursement process for these services. Behavioral care services are variably reimbursed, depending on the diagnosis, the site where care is delivered, and who is delivering the care. Thus, there is no incentive to treat "minor" cases or offer preventive services. Some researchers recruiting participants in the neighborhood offered services, but only for those cases that fit their protocol, and they were restricted by the duration of their grant. There was a tremendous need for outpatient services at all the population levels mentioned earlier. I was quite moved when a medical resident in psychiatry told me about her passion for learning about the community setting where she was doing her rotation. I was saddened, however, because the likelihood that she would end up practicing in an underserved area like northern Manhattan was slim—private practice would be more helpful in paying off her student loans.

Finally, discordance in priorities between providers and consumers was seen as a challenge to delivering quality care. For example, in my conversations with people on both sides of this dyad, I could see that while for the clinician the driving goal in treatment was stabilization and compliance, for the consumer, juggling "life" (family, work) while incorporating treatment was more important. The provider–consumer relationship is crucial in the delivery of mental health services. Racism, judgmental or insensitive staff, insensitivity for cultural differences, and lack of empathy for the population served were seen as greatly undermining treatment. But even the most culturally competent staff could face an additional challenge when there were differences in priorities between providers and consumers. The development of treatment, I found, needed to consider consumers' perceptions of their illness and the priority given to this problem in relation to other problems in their life and in their community. Treatment and follow-up were perceived as undermined if provider and consumer did not agree on the roots of the problem. For example, a provider may find that medication or group therapy is called for in a treatment plan. But if the consumer was facing problems of daily living (e.g., work schedules conflicting with therapy appointments, stigmatization related to the use of medication, housing instability or even homelessness) and these problems were not considered, then compliance with the treatment plan would be jeopardized. I recall a conversation with a young man who lived with his family of four in a two-bedroom apartment. His room had been taken over as the sewing room where his mother did piecework. It was still his room and his futon was right next to the sewing machine, but he felt that between the foot traffic of people coming to the sewing room and his frequent overnight trips to his friend's home where he felt more comfortable, he did not have a place to keep his psych medications. His friends did not know he was taking these medications, and carrying them around with him was not an option. Thus, he would constantly forget to take them.

The Northern Manhattan Mental Health Council

The Northern Manhattan Mental Health Council (NMMHC) deserves special mention since it was the only place in which all four challenge areas were addressed simultaneously. The NMMHC operated as an advising body to the Manhattan Mental Health Council, the Department of Mental Health, Mental Retardation and Alcoholism Services, and, ultimately, the State Office of Mental Health. In this body, providers and consumers were encouraged to work together at the same level. I saw this at the general meetings I attended, experienced it working side by side with both providers and consumers, and heard it in what they had to say about each other. Often, adversarial "us/theming" occurs when you put providers and consumers in each other's settings. Not so with the NMMHC. I

TABLE 12.1

Making a Difference: Mental Health Report

PROBLEM

Disparities in mental health rates and spending

Rate of mental illness hospitalization (per 1,000)
Central Harlem: 14
Manhattan: 7
New York City: 6

Rate of alcohol abuse hospitalization (per 1,000)
Central Harlem: 17
Manhattan: 5
New York City: 4

DMHRAS spending per capita
United States: $259
New York City, Chelsea/Clinton/midtown: $442
New York City, central Harlem: $88
New York City, Washington Heights/Inwood: $89

SOLUTION

Mental Health Report calls for increased commitment by local institutions

Source: New York State Department of Health (1996). Statewide Planning and Research Cooperative System. http://www.health.state.ny.us/statistics/sparcs.

always attributed this to the "thinking space" provided by the cochairs Charles Corliss and William Witherspoon and consumer chair Debra Wilson. The NMMHC became a key influence in the mental health work of Community Voices. During that time, I represented Community Voices in NMMHC meetings, collaborated in their annual legislative breakfasts, and coordinated the NMCVC efforts with theirs in the unveiling of the policy paper in the fall of 2000. Whatever impact Community Voices had on the mental health policy and programmatic agendas of our partners involved in the mental health area was due to our collaboration with the NMMHC.

The Mental Health Roundtable

A few months after the release of the policy paper *Mental Health: The Neglected Epidemic* in the late fall of 2000, the Difficult to Cover Services working group, with the support of the NMMHC, held a half-day conference to discuss recommendations and promote networking. On May 22, 2001, the Community Voices site invited members of the northern Manhattan community to a Mental Health Roundtable. Our emphasis on building relationships paid off handsomely, for that day Community Voices was able to bring together over eighty participants from all walks of life. Institutional and community-based practitioners sat side by side with consumer advocates; social workers, psychologists, and psychiatrists shared their ideas with self-made community leaders; people from Washington Heights, Inwood, and Harlem—three distinct communities that sometimes compete for the same limited resources—joined together as northern Manhattan. We even had citywide and state mental health advocates. Four discussion groups expanded on the main findings of the report: (1) Building Capacity: Assessing the Financing of Mental Health Services; (2) Prevention and Awareness: An In-depth Discussion on Stigma; (3) Service Coordination: Bridging the Gaps on the Road to Treatment; and (4) Cultural Competency: Treating the Individual in Its Context. The final summation of the findings of both the report and the roundtable was submitted to the Northern Manhattan Mental Health Council, which then presented the findings in its annual report to the New York City Department of Health.

BOX 12.2
Recommendations in the Mental Health Report

1. Prevention and Coordination of Efforts

Support with social services has been identified as a factor affecting mental health, and well-coordinated services can act as primary prevention in mental health.

Recommendations

Link mental health providers with existing community agencies that provide social services (i.e. housing, employment, child care, youth activities, services for immigrants).

Develop and support services for recently arrived immigrants that aid in diminishing stressors associated with uprooting and acculturation.

Make information on mental health and services available at all community-based agencies.

Make information on social services available at agencies providing mental health services.

2. Capacity

There is a shortage of services and trained personnel in mental health in the northern Manhattan community. Increasing the capacity of the system is a priority. The scarcity of resources is worsened by the lack of coordination between those already in place, and by suboptimal functioning of some of them due to financial instability or understaffing. Support for existing programs is vital to the strengthening of mental health services in the community. From the existing resources, school-based clinics and primary care settings have shown to be important as an access door to proper diagnosis and referral.

Recommendations

Identify and secure funding sources for existing school based clinics to sustain mental health services. Promote the creation of additional school-based clinics.

Reinforce primary care provision and access for older people.

Offer primary care providers training and technical assistance in diagnosing and treating common and uncomplicated cases.

Identify and secure continued funding for community-based organizations with ongoing mental health programs.

(Continued)

BOX 12.2 (*Continued*)

Offer training and technical assistance to informal providers of mental health (e.g., clergy in faith communities).

3. Culturally Sensitive Approaches

In northern Manhattan, support groups are deemed as a culturally appropriated way to deal with mental health problems because there is no stigma attached to these services. Users do not consider themselves as *ill*, but just having problems of daily living. This is an appropriate way to increase coverage, as it is cost-effective and can be done in community settings, in a culturally friendly environment.

Recommendations

Encourage the creation of community-based support groups as a preferred way to expand coverage in mental health.

Facilitate the increase of multicultural and multilingual staff by providing incentives. Actively promote education and training of community members.

4. Awareness

Efforts around mental illness awareness should consider using segmentation of the community (social marketing) as opposed to a generic approach. Awareness education should be extended to providers of medical care, social services, and lay personnel.

Recommendations

Address awareness campaigns to specific population groups with different concerns: adolescents, women, men, older people. Such approach may prove more useful than a uniform campaign.

Join already established citywide efforts on mental health awareness, and adapt them if necessary to our own community.

Provide information on resources in mental health and basic training in all human service settings in the community.

Following Up on Recommendations

Charlie Corliss summed up what we needed in order to follow up on rec-ommendations when he said, "I personally hoped for a large grant—2 to 3 million—to be shared by northern Manhattan CBOs [community-based organizations] to serve the uninsured and undocumented clients with pro-fessional clinical staff, since this group continues to grow yet is less and less able to get services due to the increasing rigidity of mental care." Well, we did not get the millions. In the years following the release of the report, however, several individuals in key institutions and organizations in north-ern Manhattan took our recommendations and integrated them into their work agenda.

Coordination of Services

Since the mid-1990s a group of community-based chemical dependency treatment program providers (ranging from inpatient detox to residential to outpatient clinics) had worked together under the New York State Office of Alcohol and Substance Abuse Services (OASAS). The group led a target cities initiative funded by the U.S. Center for Substance Abuse Treatment (CSAT). In March 1997 this group became a legal independent cell and called itself Target Behavioral Care (TBC). TBC membership worked dili-gently to identify protocols, estimate costs, and prepare for what at the time was to be a federally mandated Special Needs Plan (SNP) in both chemical dependency and mental health treatment. The group's goal was to survive and thrive in what was perceived as a probable "market correction" in be-havioral care. Similar to what had occurred in other states, it was expected that the demands and limits of managed care were going to force small CBOs to shut down in favor of citywide entities that could more flexibly adjust to the new, more severe marketplace.

Throughout the various phases of the New York State SNP process, TBC leadership met with a host of government and managed care rep-resentatives to assess direction. In 2001 TBC received a CSAT Capacity Expansion grant to fully operationalize its model of a complete contin-uum of behavioral care, primarily for chemical dependency treatment in high Medicaid dense communities of upper Manhattan, South Bronx, and Harlem.

By the end of the grant period in 2004, TBC had a twenty-four-hour call center linked to on-call bilingual clinicians. When consumers called for help, the clinicians linked them to their services and tracked their progress via a comprehensive software system. Much was learned, much good faith was created among community groups of like mind, and clients received service on demand. Nevertheless, TBC froze operations when the grant ended because New York State had abandoned the mental health SNP process and chemical dependency services had been carved out of the Medicaid managed care conversion process. Certain diseases or types of services—in this case chemical dependency services—are sometimes isolated from the rest of the benefits covered by an insurance product. When this happens, they may be covered by a separate vendor, in this case by a managed behavioral health care organization (e.g., Magellan Health Service, ValueOptions, United Behavioral Health). Thus, when New York carved out these services, local networks such as TBC became noncompetitive. Member agencies of the TBC network, however, continued to work informally with each other and are poised to respond to any marketplace change that would threaten the missions of the community-based organizations in favor of larger, for-profit concerns (such as the type of managed behavioral health care organizations mentioned above). The infrastructure is in place and the protocols have been worked out, so should the need or opportunity arise, the switch can be turned on.

Supporting Primary Care Providers in the Treatment
of Individuals with Mental Illness

During his participation in the committee, Roberto Lewis-Fernández met David Albert and learned about the way academic detailing was being utilized in dental settings. This model brings specialist staff to a community where the need for that particular expertise is high. The primary care provider provides information and support to the specialized provider in her or his practice to better address this need. Lewis-Fernández adapted this model and paired up a group of local primary care providers with a traveling team of psychiatrists who provided case consultation and medication management on site. This project was supported by Community Voices in its inception by submitting various research and service grants to implement and test the model. The model was later funded by a series of foundations and finally by a research grant from National Institute of Mental Health.

Mental Illness in the African American Community

In collaboration with the New York City Metro chapter of the National Alliance on Mental Illness, Community Voices brought together more than two hundred residents to dialogue and network with faith-based professionals, health care providers, community leaders, family members, and consumers to address mental illness in the African American community. This event, entitled "Heal the Mind, Restore the Spirit: Mental Health Recognition and Recovery in the African-American Community," was held on September 24, 2005, at the Abyssinian Baptist Church in Harlem. The conference included a series of dynamic workshops by representatives from the Stay Strong Foundation, the New York City Department of Health and Mental Hygiene Office of Consumer Affairs, the Judah International Christian Center, the American Psychiatric Foundation, and the cochair of the Steering Committee to Reduce Disparities in Access to Psychiatric Care.

National Alliance on Mental Illness New York City Metro Board member Karen Gormandy talked about her experience at the conference: "As the mother of a child with mental illness, I cannot stress the importance of networking through events like this conference. You may arrive confused, isolated and possibly desperate, but you will leave with concrete information, guidance, and the support of your community—able to address mental health issues in your family. Most importantly, you will discover that you are not alone, and that the struggle can be won."

Mental Health Treatment in Primary Care Settings

The formation of the Difficult to Cover Services working group, the resulting activities, and the report together served as a catalyst for institutional policy changes. The integration of the collaborative model of mental health care in the ambulatory care centers of the hospital was one such change. As of today, the Ambulatory Clinics of New York Presbyterian Hospital in northern Manhattan and the Thelma Adair Clinic in Harlem have adopted this model and have made access to mental health services a possibility for hundreds of community residents. Most health care settings take care of physical health (minus oral health, sadly), with the extent of their mental health care limited to medication management for milder cases of mental illness. The collaborative model employed by the above-mentioned facilities pairs up mental health professionals (psychiatrists, psychologists, clinical social workers) in the same setting to provide, in addition to the medication management, an array of individual and group counseling modalities.

Impact beyond Northern Manhattan

The Difficult to Cover Services working group provided an opportunity for health leaders and community members to collaborate and develop a unified (and hence, stronger) voice to inform policies that were undermining access to care for community residents. One of the key recommendations made by the Community Voices policy paper was for parity in the reimbursement of mental health services with other health services. The report served as a tool for working group members, Community Voices staff, and other community leaders to participate in discussions concerning mental health parity with statewide policy makers. The report prompted other community collaboratives to focus on the issue, and it supported the efforts of statewide advocacy groups committed to mental health parity. As a result, members of the working group, as well as Community Voices staff members, became intricately engaged in statewide and citywide discussions about the issue.

Such statewide discussions led to new New York State legislation. In January 2007 Governor Elliot Spitzer signed into law a bill requiring that commercial insurance policies cover mental health services similar to the way they cover costs for other health treatment. New York now joins the other twenty-two states that have parity laws. The new law should pave the way to improved care for those covered by commercial insurance. There is still more work to be accomplished for those covered by Medicare. However, this new law will provide a model for all payors to follow.

The Difficult to Cover Services working group and the ensuing mental health report also served as a critical vehicle to mobilize community resources toward improving mental health access. The leadership that emerged and the collective voice prompted change within organizations and institutions, and, more important, it allowed community leaders and consumers to become active participants in the efforts to inform policy changes that would eliminate barriers to mental health care.

Many of the individuals who worked on developing the report went on to make significant contributions in improving access to mental health care in northern Manhattan. I am very happy to call many of them my mentors. Being part of the Northern Manhattan Community Voices Collaborative shaped the rest of my career and proved to me that ugly ducklings could reap beautiful results.

Postscript

I wish I had a happy ending for the Northern Manhattan Mental Health Council, but I do not. When New York City transitioned from a two-branch system (mental health and health) to the current Department of Health and Mental Hygiene, the Mental Health Councils across the five boroughs were disbanded. These councils existed thanks to the independence that the mental health branch (Department of Mental Health, Mental Retardation and Alcoholism Services) afforded. The merger effectively eliminated the mechanism through which consumers and providers could advocate, inform policy makers, and effect change. No alternative mechanisms have been reinstituted.

Note

1. The Community Scholars Program was an NMCVC-funded program administered through the School of Public Health. Its purpose was to recruit a cadre of individuals from the community with an interest in community-based work while pursuing their master's degree.

References

Lewis-Fernández, R., et al. (2005). Depression in U.S. Hispanics: Diagnostic and management considerations in family practice. *Journal of the American Board of Family Practice* 18, no. 4: 282–96.

National Alliance on Mental Illness website. http://www.nami.org.

Northern Manhattan Community Voices Collaborative (2001). *Mental health: The neglected epidemic, a report of the Difficult to Cover Services work group.* New York: Columbia University, Center for Community Health Partnerships.

Pear, R. (2008). House approves bill on mental health parity. *New York Times.* March 6.

Scholarly Publishing and Academic Resources Coalition (SPARC) data. (1996).

U.S. Department of Health and Human Services (1999). *Mental health: A report of the surgeon general—executive summary.* Rockville, Md.: U.S. Department of Health and Human Services, Substance Abuse and Mental Health Services Administration, Center for Mental Health Services, National Institutes of Health, National Institute of Mental Health.

U.S. Public Health Service (1999). *The surgeon general's call to action to prevent suicide.* Washington, D.C.

13

The Thelma C. Davidson Adair Medical/Dental Center

ALLAN J. FORMICOLA

> Ultimately it took unwavering commitment by the individuals who be-
> lieved in the vision to establish this freestanding primary care facility
> to get it up and running. Slowly and with determination, those indi-
> viduals slogged through a myriad of seemingly irresolvable problems
> to turn this vision into reality.

Establishing a free-standing primary care clinic in the middle of Harlem is not a decision to be taken lightly, especially in the mid-1990s when the country had yet to embrace primary care as the best way to get on top of the nation's health care problems. Yet, that is just what the Northern Manhat-tan Community Voices Collaborative did when it acted upon a recommen-dation from the Community DentCare planning group (chapter 11). Dur-ing the planning process for DentCare, the Harlem planning group was pleased that children would become the target group for beginning dental programs in the public schools, but they asked for some consideration for older Harlem residents who had been long overlooked. The planning group, led by Dennis Mitchell, persuaded the NMCVC Difficult to Cover Services working group that this recommendation should be taken seriously. This decision greatly complicated DentCare's original premise that emphasiz-ing preventive and early treatment for children was the best way to develop a community-wide or population-based intervention to improve the oral health of northern Manhattan residents.

However, it was true that Harlem had more older residents than did other sections of Manhattan, and that they were often overlooked. Clearly, the clergy whose congregations were composed mainly of older people in-fluenced the Harlem DentCare planning group. One of the members of that planning group was Thelma Adair, a long-time Harlem activist on social issues on behalf of the Harlem community. She was also the wife of the late Reverend Adair, who became pastor at the Mount Morris Baptist Church in the early 1940s. He and Thelma had moved to Harlem from South Carolina and intended to stay for only a year or two, but fifty years later she was still hard at work—at the age of 80—and fully engaged in the problems of the underserved in Harlem. Thelma Adair, a woman of great talents, eventually earned a doctorate degree in education from Teachers College, Columbia University. However, she never lost her spirit and compassion for social justice issues, and she became a major force in the long process of building the center named for her. Her fingerprints are all over the effort to bring the new center into fruition, and the building of the center is as much a story about Thelma Adair as it is about the NMCVC.

The NMCVC working group for this effort was led by me, then the dean of the dental school, and Tom Morris. Morris was a long-standing Columbia University Medical Center leader who served in a number of leadership roles, including president of Presbyterian Hospital, interim dean of the College of Physicians and Surgeons, and vice president of the Columbia Health Science Schools. We both recognized the difficulties of building a primary care facility in Harlem. The Health and Hospitals Corporation, the public hospital system in New York City, basically had a monopoly on the health system in Harlem. Harlem Hospital was one of the original partners of the NMCVC and affiliated with the Columbia University College of Physicians and Surgeons and the College of Dental Medicine. Even so, the hospital and their central Health and Hospitals Corporation administration looked with suspicion on the idea of the NMCVC building a health center in Harlem—even a small one as envisioned by the Harlem NMCVC planning committee. Morris and I recognized the many forces at work in Harlem and Columbia University that could and would create formidable barriers toward moving forward with this recommendation.

After meeting Thelma Adair and visiting with one of the congregations in Harlem, I was convinced that while it made sense from a community-wide intervention point of view to target just children for an oral health care initiative, it made equal sense from a humanistic point of view to do something for older people in Harlem who had been overlooked and given little to no consideration in targeted efforts to improve their health year in and year out. In my role as dean of the School of Dental and Oral Surgery (now known as the College of Dental Medicine) and the primary investigator for the NMCVC project, I endorsed the recommendation to move the planning forward for an oral health initiative for older people in Harlem. In looking back, it was hard to conceive in 1998 that this decision would lead to a complicated set of problems, which would play out over an entire decade. Barriers were everywhere in carrying out this endeavor— from regulatory barriers to financial, and from institutional to personal.

The development of the Thelma C. Davidson Adair Medical/Dental Center in central Harlem is a microcosm of the challenges for the entire primary care system in underserved communities. However, while this chapter will describe some of these challenges, the one big lesson that stands out in reflecting on this part of the NMCVC story is that ultimately it took unwavering commitment by the individuals who believed in the vision to establish this freestanding primary care facility to get it up and running. Slowly and with determination, those individuals slogged through a myriad of seemingly irresolvable problems to turn this vision into reality.

This chapter first asks what was the vision for the Adair Center that captured the attention of many individuals over the past decade, and then

TABLE 13.1

Making a Difference: The Adair Center

PROBLEMS

Most common health complaint in Harlem: problems with teeth and gums
Overcrowded clinics short on ambiance
Elderly dental care overlooked
One-third of those with dental problems did not seek care

SOLUTION

"Park Avenue"-type facility that serves patients in a dignified manner

RESULTS (2006–2007)

Total visits: 8,414
Dental visits: 5,559
Total medical visits: 2,855
Total medicaid visits: 64%
Total medicare visits: 3%
Commercial insurance: 19%
Self-pay: 14%
Users at or below poverty level: 80%
African American users: 70%

Sources: Zabos (2008); Adair Center records.

what are the barriers that had to be overcome. Since I have been at the center of the story since its inception, it will be told as seen through my eyes. My commitment, matched throughout by that of Thelma Adair and others, clearly demonstrates the old saying, "Where there is a will there is a way." So, what was this vision?

The Vision: A "Park Avenue" Practice

The citizens of Harlem have largely been served by a public hospital system, including hospitals and clinics dispersed throughout the community. Additionally, several community-based organizations (some of long standing) had established clinics in Harlem. Generally, most clinics in underserved communities are overcrowded, have long waiting times for the patients, and lack what could be called a private practice ambience. Patients become accustomed to the idea of sitting and waiting to see the doctor and being treated according to a herd mentality. The Adair Center, however, was based on the idea that Harlem citizens should have a facility that is patient friendly to older people as well as all others who use the facility and that operates like a "Park Avenue" practice. The facility should look more like an upscale private practice, work mainly on an appointment basis, and treat individuals with the same courtesy as patients receive on Park Avenue, even though the facility would serve largely a Medicaid-reimbursed population. We believed that those who sought care should have a primary care home, and one where the physicians and dentists were familiar and responsible for their overall care. We realized that this type of center would be difficult to deliver on, but the vision for it still inspires those who work in the Adair Center. In Thelma Adair's words, it's "kind of fun to go over and to see people able to have an appointment. And wait a few minutes, and go in, and not spend all day just waiting to see if I can get an appointment. That says something about what you think about this population. Your time is valuable, too."

Dennis Mitchell, a recently hired full-time dentist faculty member of the College of Dental Medicine, had a central role in the Adair Center story. Mitchell completed his dental degree at the Howard University Dental School and came to Harlem Hospital for his general dentistry residency training. Here, he was put under the wing of James McIntosh, director of Harlem Hospital's Dental Service and a close colleague of mine. In addition to his dental training and while a resident at the hospital, Mitchell completed a special program (see also the epilogue) in public health at Columbia's Mailman School of Public Health. This additional training in public health provided Mitchell with exceptional preparation, and, as indicated above, he was selected to head the Harlem DentCare planning group. As a young African American dental practitioner as well as an astute public health practitioner, he was well aware of the poor state of health of many older people. A highly sensitive and dedicated individual, Mitchell took the first concrete step in moving the Adair Center from dream to reality: he discovered an important building in Harlem in which to create the center.

Finding a Space

To better understand the oral health problems of older people, Mitchell conducted a survey of those living in a senior citizens' center in Harlem, the Mannie L. Wilson Center. While conducting the survey, Mitchell, whose personality is extremely outgoing, got to know the superintendent of the building. One day the superintendent showed him space on the basement level that had been put aside for a small medical facility when the building was transformed from the Syndenham Hospital to a senior citizens' center. The closure of the Syndenham Hospital in 1979 had become a major community issue and coincidentally touched on some of the players in the Adair Center story. James McIntosh, then head of the Medical Board of the hospital, was among those who had locked themselves in the building to prevent the hospital's closure. After a long standoff between the hospital staff and the police, McIntosh and several others were jailed briefly for refusing the order to leave the building. Thelma Adair also came to see this location as symbolic as she recalled the uproar in the community over the closure of the facility. The closure, she explains, rallied the community against what it believed was the abandonment of the dire needs of the Harlem community. Recently, former New York City mayor Ed Koch, in an interview with a *New York Times* reporter, expressed misgivings about his decision to close the Sydenham Hospital. Koch said, "In retrospect there was such a psychological attachment to Sydenham because black doctors couldn't get into other hospitals. It was the psychological attachment that I violated. That was uncaring of me" (Roberts 2009). Some thirty years later, Mitchell brought me to see this space.

At first glance, it looked rather small, dingy, unappealing, and inappropriate for the concept of the facility I had in mind. And then, in a twist of fate, everything changed. One day, Mitchell and I were talking about how difficult it would be to turn this space into the center we envisioned because it would be too cramped. The superintendent of the building happened to overhear our conversation and said that beyond the back wall lay a vast amount of unused space that could be added to the existing space. By this point in the planning process, the facility plan called for not only a dental facility but also a medical facility. This vision took form because a survey of the senior citizens had shown that they had much neglected dental disease coupled with major general health problems—a scenario that thus required a collaborative facility between medicine and dentistry to provide good, comprehensive care in one place. Mitchell and I took one look at this space and immediately realized its exciting potential. The boarded up windows in what could become the waiting room could be opened to let natural light pour in. With a good architect's plan, the entire block of space could be converted into the "Park Avenue"-like medical/dental center we both envisioned. Thelma Adair recalls, "We almost gave up because we couldn't find the space. But the janitor just happened to be there. It really makes you believe in the Cinderella story." But the story was far from over.

Red Tape and Greenbacks

Little did we realize that gaining the right to build the center in this space would involve the federal Department of Housing and Urban Development (HUD), who owned the building. This difficulty emerged only slowly, since the building was managed by a local community group known as the West Harlem Group. The West Harlem Group was headed up by Donald Notice, who quickly realized the benefits of converting this unused space into an asset for the building and a good service for the Harlem community. The Mannie L. Wilson building is strategically located on 124th Street and Manhattan Avenue, one block south of the 125th Street heart of Harlem and just one block south from a major subway stop. Elated at the location, the history of the facility, and the willingness of Donald Notice and his staff to rent the space, I proceeded to delve into the financial issues while Mitchell worked on the facility plan.

I realized that none of the funds awarded by the W. K. Kellogg Foundation for the NMCVC could be used for building facilities. I also realized that the College of Dental Medicine that I headed did not have the resources to build the center, and that the university expected those interested in developing such service programs to raise outside funds for such purposes. However, even with those caveats, the leadership at Columbia University encouraged me to pursue the plan because the creation of the medical/dental center would be an expression of the university's good neighborness in the Harlem community. The university wished to demonstrate a positive relationship with Harlem, as there has been a long history of antagonism between the two. In addition, the university was thinking ahead toward expansion of its campus into west Harlem, not far from where the Adair Center would be located. All that was needed was the funding to turn the idea into reality. For this, another character in the story, the Primary Care Development Corporation (PCDC), became the means.

Aware that the corporation was set up by the state and the city to assist in the development of primary care facilities, I contacted Ronda Kotelchuck, executive director of the PCDC, and we arranged to meet. Kotelchuck told me that PCDC provides a combination of grant and loan funds to build or expand primary care facilities in the city. She noted that PCDC had backed about twenty separate primary care facilities in various locations but had not found a group to work with in Harlem. By the time our meeting was over, Kotelchuck realized that the center I described might just be the Harlem facility that PCDC could fund. PCDC soon provided us with a small grant for facility design, which we used to hire an architect through a competitive application process.

The architect took the concept of a "Park Avenue"-like practice into account and transformed the basement space of the Mannie Wilson Tower building into a pleasing and efficient medical and dental office environment. The price tag for the construction was estimated to be $2.6 million, and the PCDC came through with a $400,000 grant and a PCDC-backed bank loan of $2 million. I needed to raise the remaining $200,000 from a previous university loan to improve the clinical facilities of the College of Dental Medicine. The commitment from PCDC allowed the plan to move forward toward final planning, but again the story was not over. First came a battle with HUD, which would only approve the application to convert the unused space into a medical facility if the facility limited its patient list to the approximately two hundred patients living in the Mannie L. Wilson Towers.

The financial plan required the facility to be self-supporting after a start-up period, but the limited patient base HUD permitted would not be sufficient to support the anticipated expenses. Nevertheless, the New York HUD officials were adamant: HUD policy simply did not permit those outside of a HUD facility to be treated. Enter Ivy Fairchild, the assistant vice president for community affairs at the Medical Center, and Charles Rangel, the long-term congressman from Harlem. Together, they were able to put the case before federal HUD officials, arguing that important community benefit would accrue from allowing this facility to treat not only the residents of the building but also those living in the surrounding community. Finally, after a year of back and forth and a public airing of the question, HUD issued a change in policy. It would allow the West Harlem Group to negotiate a long-term lease with Columbia University Health Care Inc., the appropriate university entity behind the NMCVC. As I reflect on this period, Ivy Fairchild especially stands out as another of the committed individuals who bought into the vision. She had the tenacity and the fortitude to move the agenda forward at both the federal and state level and change the minds of key officials to permit the dream to move forward.

A twenty-year lease was negotiated with the West Harlem Group. With funding from the PCDC and the College of Dental Medicine, the construction began with an estimated completion in 2000 or early 2001. At this point, I realized that the finances of primary care facilities were the critical element but that the facility would treat a large proportion of Medicaid patients. This meant that the community residents to be served would not have the resources available to pay for medical and dental care that those patients being treated in "Park Avenue" practices have at their disposal. I further realized that paying off a $2 million loan would be burdensome to the center and that sooner rather than later a new source of funding was necessary to pay off the loan if the facility was to be able to pay its own costs. Given the facility's key location in central Harlem, an area of interest to many state agencies, it seemed appropriate to turn to the state for assistance. Thelma Adair volunteered to assist. She recognized that if this new center was to come to fruition additional funding was needed, and that the community itself would need to ask for it rather than the university.

Senior Citizens Go to Albany

Working with Dennis Mitchell, Thelma Adair brought a group of senior citizens to Albany to request funding for the facility. That trip to Albany is a fond memory for Adair. She recalls that early on the morning of the trip, she and her team of seniors met at the medical center. Mitchell arrived with donuts in hand and everyone loaded into a small van. Spirits were high in the ride up to Albany as this group of seniors was committed to finding a solution for their oral health needs. Most of them had lost their teeth and had no dentures to replace them. All you had to do is look at them and you could see their need for care. This became an asset in asking their representatives in Albany to help get this facility off the ground.

Sitting in the back of a conference room loaned to Adair and her friends, I marveled at the ability of the seniors to present the case to the many representatives and their staff who came by to see them. Usually it is the other way around—constituents need to visit the offices of their representatives one by one, which generally is a time-consuming process. However, the word spread quickly that here was a group of seniors from Harlem that had come up to Albany, and the representatives and their staff members decided in deference to them to reverse the process by coming to see them. There was no need for Dennis Mitchell or me to say a word. We were all in high spirits again on the ride back to Manhattan because we felt the importance of our mission was understood. "The ride from Harlem to Albany became an opportunity for us to get to know each other in a different way . . . like peeling back the many layers of an onion and each layer has a flavor," recalls Thelma Adair. "The ride in and of itself became an important part of the whole. . . . there was constantly a willingness to let go of the [acrimoniousness of] the past and to search for other ways of doing it."

The van ride was the opening salvo for state support, but it took the next five years, many subsequent trips to Albany, and the support of the university president to realize the state aid that would pay off the construction loan.

It appeared that with many of the challenges successfully confronted, the time was right to give the facility a name. We unanimously and enthusiastically supported naming the facility for Thelma Adair. James McIntosh joined me in hosting a lunch for Adair at a restaurant in Harlem. She was thrilled with the idea but insisted that the facility carry her full name—Thelma C. Davidson Adair—because it recognized and honored all the elements of her family heritage of long life and struggle for equality. The marquee for the facility says "The Thelma C. Davidson Adair Medical/ Dental Center of Columbia University Health Care, Inc." Thelma likes to say that she is very pleased when her friends and others stop her on the street and say that they like "her" facility.

Opening the Doors

By the late spring of 2001 the construction was completed; however, there were no start-up funds yet identified to open the doors. The financial plan required several years of subsidy to get the facility up and running. The reimbursement rate could not support the start-up costs for the physician, dentist, and support staff and the operational costs, including the payback costs of the loan. It was expected to cost about $1 million to subsidize the start-up costs while the patient base slowly rose to about 12,000–14,000 visits per year. And then, in the midst of trying to raise the necessary funding, 9/11 happened. Getting attention for this facility became exceedingly difficult. However, again fortune intervened. The W. K. Kellogg senior program officer in charge of the NMCVC national program, Henrie Treadwell, was on one of her site visits of the NMCVC. I recall vividly sitting in one of my meetings with her lamenting the fact that this wonderful facility was still empty because we did not have the necessary start-up funds. Sometimes you get lucky and this was the day! Henrie Treadwell realized that this facility was one of the NMCVC's key initiatives in Harlem. She knew that the Kellogg Foundation was making funds available to its grantees to off-set hardships that came up after 9/11. With her assistance and support, the Kellogg Foundation made available to us a $1 million start-up grant that allowed us to open the doors.

The new grant did not reassure all of the skeptics, both within and outside the university, that the new center would be successful in achieving its financial plan of self-sufficiency. After twenty-three years of service, I completed my deanship of the College of Dental Medicine and, in October 2001, was able to devote more time and effort to making the center successful. I enlisted Stephen Marshall, now an associate dean in the College of Dental Medicine. Marshall was an excellent administrator who was able to navigate the complex university processes necessary to operate the facility. He oversaw the hiring of the professional and support staff and the budget process. Since half of the facility was devoted to medical care, Robert Lewy, an associate dean in the medical school who joined me in establishing a new center at Columbia, the Center for Community Health Partnerships, agreed to supervise the medical care provided by the physicians. Catherine Chan, the onsite administrator, and the new center's financial officer completed the team, and a regular oversight process was put into place to move the Adair Center into a fully functional facility.

Keeping the Doors Open

In the grand scheme of things and in relation to the major medical and dental facilities operated by the College of Dental Medicine and the College of Physicians and Surgeons faculty practices, the Adair Center was small in size; however, its strategic location in central Harlem and its special mission attracted unusual attention. The dedication of the professional and support staff to the mission also continually motivated the management team to work even harder to make sure the facility was successful. However, after the first full year of operation, it became apparent that over the long term and after the start-up funds were spent, the facility would be unable to support itself, given the high census of Medicaid patients, the relatively low reimbursement rate, and the need to pay back a $2 million loan.

I had not given up on obtaining state funds for the construction and continued to pursue that objective, working with community leaders and university officials. A number of the locally elected members of the State Assembly actively supported and assisted in this action, including Keith Wright and Adriano Espaillat. Assemblyman Herman D. ("Denny") Farrell recognized the need to find state funding for the facility. Church leaders also assisted. I recall a visit to the Adair Center with Reverend Calvin Butts of the Abyssinian Baptist Church, who was considering supporting the request for state funds. He came to see the facility, and what a surprise he received as he walked along: he recognized one of his congregants receiving dental care. What was so remarkable about this incident was that he recognized this congregant just by seeing the back of her head as she sat waiting for care in a dental chair. He not only recognized her but knew her by name. After meeting the professional staff and seeing the level of care being provided, Reverend Butts too became one of the individuals who advocated for state funds. The practical and symbolic value of the Adair Center resonated with anyone who had a sense of history.

The university budget officials stressed the importance of contingency planning given the weak finances of the facility. The Adair Center was not the only primary care center struggling in Harlem. Two small facilities operated by St. Luke's Hospital closed, demonstrating the difficulty of operating health facilities in that community. The health centers able to survive, designated as Federally Qualified Health Centers (FQHCs), were receiving an enhanced reimbursement rate for the care they provided to Medicaid patients and an annual grant from the federal government to help provide indigent care. The Adair Center could not qualify for such designation. Even when the state finally provided the $2 million for the construction, it took an additional university loan of $1 million to subsidize the operating budget as the original $1 million Kellogg Foundation start-up grant had been expended.

One of the contingency plans for the Adair Center, therefore, was to partner with another existing health center, ideally an FQHC. Torn between the options to partner or to call it quits during its fifth year of operating, the Adair Center management team took on the task of identifying a partner. Stephen Marshall recommended that Heritage Health and Housing Inc., a community-based FQHC, could be such a partner. He noted that if the Adair Center had their reimbursement rate it would break even. But there was still $1 million in debt owed to the university for the facility. The question became: would Heritage, which wanted to acquire the facility as an expansion site to their existing health facility on nearby 144th Street and Amsterdam Avenue, be able to carry the costs of paying off the $1 million loan? Initially, Heritage believed that they could do just that; however, subsequently the Health Resources Service Administration, the federal agency that oversees FQHC facilities, concluded that they could not.

It now became incumbent on the leadership in the Medical Center to take the next step. No one wanted to see the Adair Center close, and everyone believed for the long-term good a partnership with Heritage was desirable, but that meant forgiving the outstanding university loan of $1 million. Essentially, this was a win-win situation for everyone and would have been a turn-key operation for Heritage. Heritage would get a wonderful, fully equipped facility worth over $2.5 million with no debt. The Adair Center was handling about eight thousand patient visits a year. After reevaluating the various options, the executive vice president of the Columbia University

Medical Center decided to forgive the loan, making it possible to complete the transfer of the facility to Heritage. However, after almost two years of working with Heritage, the deal fell through. In May 2008 Jorge Abreu, president and chief executive officer of Heritage, called to tell me that his board would no longer go along with acquiring the Adair Center. Shortly after the negotiations fell through, Abreu left his position.

In the summer of 2008 the dean of the College of Dental Medicine, Ira Lamster, stepped into this void. He determined that the Adair Center would make a good setting in which to educate dental students and felt that it was in the college's best interests to take responsibility for the center. This was good news, as the center would remain firmly in the hands of Columbia University, which had many interests in keeping the facility open. However, the faculty of the College of Dental Medicine was not able to see the benefit of educating students at the Adair Center, and the dean had to withdraw his offer. This left us high and dry, so to speak. We knew that the university's plans called for expanding its campus just west of the Thelma Adair Center into what is called Manhattanville. It would be beneficial for the university to continue to operate the center to help reduce community opposition to the expansion plan and show itself as a good citizen of the community. However, the negative financial bottom line became an issue that the university and/or its medical and dental schools were no longer able or willing to support.

The Columbia University Medical Center administration established a task force to decide what to do about continuing the operation of the center. In December 2008 they concluded that due to financial concerns, the center would close at the end of June 2009 if a new entity could not be found to take over ownership. Along with my colleagues Stephen Marshall and Robert Lewy, I worried that the closing of the center would be a vivid sign to the Harlem community that the university did not really care about it after all. We were concerned that a wonderful primary care facility for the community would be lost.

Fortunately, in May 2009 Stephen Marshall found others who were willing to consider taking responsibility for the Adair Center. The Ryan Health Center, a well-respected FQHC that had other facilities operating in Manhattan, saw the value of adding the Adair Center to its network. Marshall negotiated all of the outstanding issues for the Ryan Center to take ownership and operate the Adair facility so that there would be no disruption of service when the university pulled out at the end of June. On

July 1, 2009, the Ryan Center took over the Adair Center as its new owner. Importantly, the Ryan Center understood the significance of keeping the center's name as the Thelma C. Davidson Adair Center, and in a meeting with representatives of Columbia and Thelma Adair prior to the handoff its leaders expressed their desire to do so. As longtime providers of care to underserved populations, the Ryan Center understands the connections of its facilities to the community it serves, and keeping Thelma Adair's name on the center is an expression of such understanding.

One Big Dilemma

Although the Adair Center is not in the Columbia family any more, it is gratifying that the story can end on a happy note. But the story demonstrates the larger problems of the health care system in the United States. While many policy makers involved in health care speak about the importance of primary care, the system does not promote it or have policies that allow primary care centers to thrive in the United States. Yes, the eight hundred or so Federally Qualified Health Care Centers have ways to cushion the harsh financial realities of operating a primary care center, but those benefits do not extend to an unaffiliated center such as the Adair Center. Stephen Marshall pointed out that if the Adair Center had the same reimbursement rate as an FQHC and an annual grant to support the provision of care to low-income populations, at its current volume of patients and visits it would have been financially viable. However, that was not the case. The annual volume of visits would have had to grow more rapidly, to 12,000 to 14,000, in order for the reimbursement rate we were receiving to cover costs. That was not happening. Why we were not able to more rapidly add patients to those we were attracting can fill another volume. Suffice it to say that it was probably a combination of factors, from complicated university management systems to rapid turnover of the critical professional staff, and from inefficient patient throughput to complex credentialing processes. With the experience of the last decade, it is very clear to me why so few wish to take on the challenge of attempting to improve our health care system by planning and operating primary care centers.

The long-range solution for primary care facilities in low-income communities will require broader thinking on the part of policy makers to encourage others to take on the challenges. Unless policies at the national and local levels are developed to facilitate primary care, the U.S. health system will not reach those citizens in dire need of basic health care. We will continue with a have and have-not system.

On the other hand, by examining the experiences of primary care centers such as the Adair Center, policy makers could begin to find solutions to the issues of bringing care to the underserved. So, I think it is ultimately helpful to put the Adair Center into the broader context of the goals and objectives of the Community Voices national program. Community Voices was the Kellogg Foundation's instrument for helping local communities shore up the fragile safety net serving underserved populations. The NMCVC had a far-reaching set of plans to do that in northern Manhattan. Each of the NMCVC projects was designed ultimately to build community capacity to improve the safety net. The Adair Center was one of the many projects, and the NMCVC served to motivate those in the university concerned about service issues to find creative ways to work with the community, secure funding, and use appropriate university resources to develop the new center.

Here is what Thelma Adair has said about the experience: "For many years [Syndenham Hospital] represented the denial of services to racial and economic groupings." But in the Adair Center "we have an opportunity to create a facility that is open to all." She went on to say that for her, it was "a continuation of the [civil rights] struggle that made this even more significant to me . . . the joy was showing how the strengths of such diverse groups and persons could be used to create such a positive resource for an underserved community. . . . I think it gives dignity to everybody." Upon learning of the university's plans to close the center at the end of June 2009, Adair expressed regret that the university had missed the opportunity to continue what she believed was a wonderful partnership with the community. However, she joined with us to help create the proper environment for the Ryan Center to take over. Upon reflection, I realized that her belief in this primary care center located just one block south of 125th Street and the Apollo Theater, the heart of Harlem, the support of so many of the political leaders, as well as the commitment of my colleagues Stephen Marshall and Robert Lewy, was what carried us through the difficult and complex issues associated with this NMCVC project. It takes strong leadership and vision to successfully negotiate the barriers to such an endeavor.

References

Centers for Medicare and Medicaid Services website. http://www.cms.hhs.gov/center/fqhc.asp.

Grumbach, K., and T. Bodenheimer (2002). A primary care home for Americans: Putting the house in order. *JAMA* 288, no. 7: 889–93.

New York City Department of Health and Mental Hygiene (2006). Community health profiles. http://www.nyc.gov/html/doh/html/data/data.shtml

Primary Care Development Corporation in collaboration with New York State Health Foundation (2009). The deteriorating financial health of New York State's health centers. March.

Roberts, Sam (2009). Koch makes his peace and dares to look ahead. An interview with former mayor Ed Koch. *New York Times*, March 1.

Zabos, G. P., et al. (2008). Lack of oral health care for adults in Harlem: A hidden crisis. *American Journal of Public Health* 98, no. S1: S102–5.

Part V

Summing Up and Scaling Up

This part summarizes the work of the Northern Manhattan Community Voices Collaborative in bringing together the academic center and the community, and vice versa. It also presents a plan for scaling up prevention successes to the national level.

[14]

Summing Up

ALLAN J. FORMICOLA and LOURDES HERNÁNDEZ-CORDERO

This chapter is entitled "Summing Up" because we thought it important to reflect on the lessons we learned in order to put them into perspective for the broader application we propose in the final chapter, "Scaling Up."

To recap the broad picture: the W. K. Kellogg Foundation's initiative, Community Voices: Health Care for the Underserved, was created to set up learning laboratories where communities address local health issues and improve the safety net for their populations, and where strategies would emerge that could be used effectively on a broader scale. Thirteen sites around the nation were funded with grants that required them to improve the general medical and oral health safety net in their communities. In New York, the Northern Manhattan Community Voices Collaborative was selected for funding by the Kellogg Foundation. It exemplifies a partnership among a major research university (Columbia University School of Dental and Oral Surgery, now called the College of Dental Medicine); a large, community-based organization (Alianza Dominicana) located in Washington Heights, a mainly Latino community in northern Manhattan; and a community-based health care provider (Harlem Hospital Dental Service).

The writing of this book has provided us the opportunity to reflect on the challenges facing the collaborative and draw lessons learned from its work over the past decade. In the beginning of the book, we asked whether the large institutions in northern Manhattan could successfully collaborate with their surrounding community to advance two important goals: to ascertain the capacity in the community to educate itself about health and build on it as needed, and to sustain pilots and projects begun.

Then, we set out the four NMCVC initiatives. First, it would enroll eligible individuals into existing publicly funded health insurance plans. Second, it would develop health promotion and disease prevention programs. Third, it would plan and develop a new affordable insurance product for uninsured individuals. And fourth, it would address the mental and oral health needs of the population. Parts 2–4 describe the detailed stories behind these four initiatives. Below we summarize some of the major accomplishments of the NMCVC regarding them.

- 1,500 community health workers were trained; they have become the bridge between the institutions, community-based organizations, and the residents and make the health system work for the people.
- 30,000 eligible adults and children were enrolled in health plans, opening up access to care for those previously unable to obtain it. Hospitalization statistics were reduced, from 21 percent to 9 percent, for those participants in the Asthma Basics for Children initiative.
- The vaccination rate for the sample group of 6,990 children in the Start Right program increased from 63 percent (below the national and New York City rate) to 96.8 percent, surpassing the New York City rate and the goal set in Healthy People 2010.
- The tobacco cessation clinic had an improved quit rate, from 24 percent of those treated to 68 percent, demonstrating that the bio-psycho-social approach works in a low socioeconomic community.
- The use of the hospital's emergency department was reduced by 95 percent for frequent users enrolled in the CARE program.
- A primary care medical and dental center was established in central Harlem, providing for 8,000 patient visits a year, with the capacity to expand to providing for 12,000–14,000 patient visits a year.
- Dental prevention programs in eight public schools in northern Manhattan were established, along with a mobile van providing care to Head Start children and older people.

- The W. K. Kellogg Foundation funding of $5.5 million was leveraged to over $45 million.

Achieving these successes was not easy, and we faced many challenges both large and small. In reflection, there were three main challenges that caused us to continually reassess the way we were managing the collaborative:

- *Developing a workable organization structure and staffing infrastructure* that would interact between institution and community in a mutually respectful way. Selecting members of committees who had knowledge of existing initiatives that could be built upon and of the cultural norms of the community and institutions, and who had the authority to speak for their respective entities, required the buy-in of the top leadership, which was not always easy to secure. Committees required paid staff that would follow up on initiatives, and it was not easy to always provide the staff the committee members perceived to be sufficient.

- *Burnout and keeping up interest over a long period of time.* In the initial years the excitement of the initiative and being selected as a funded site helped to sustain the momentum of the collaborative. To this followed a period of developing a trusted "brand name" that opened the doors to establish new relationships. When the goals of the program shifted from piloting community- and institution-based projects to policy matters, however, interest by the broader community waned since less of the NMCVC energies went into running specific community-based projects.

- *Communicating results of the initiatives along the way to the community at large.* Community forums and awards programs for partnership accomplishments aided in communicating results, but a clear sense of which audiences needed to be reached and a precise dissemination plan were not in place. These two elements would have enhanced the ability of the NMCVC to communicate more effectively and obtain necessary feedback.

One of our failures in setting up the NMCVC and its goals was that we paid little to no attention to the impact the projects would have on the missions, goals, and financial interests of the entities who would need to sustain them. However, we did understand from the start that whatever programs we field tested would need to be adopted by established entities because our overarching goal was to shore up the existing safety net, not establish a new entity. It became apparent in analyzing successes and failures that when a project or program did not fit in well with the existing mission, it was liable to fail. It also is important to think through the financial implications of initiatives to decide whether it is possible to take them on. On the other hand, unless one is prepared to think broader than the status quo, we will not advance the current system to be more responsive to the needs of the public. Institutions and community-based organizations have to be willing to consider stretching their mission and convincing funding sources that the advances their programs can make are ones that will gain their support. In moving forward we realize that one of the keys to sustainability is that some element of the existing mission or work agenda of all partners needs to be reflected in the collaboration. Once that is in place, the stretching we propose can happen.

The capacity of the community to educate itself has been advanced, for example, by the Center for Health Promotion and Education that Alianza established and the hundreds of community health workers trained who work directly with residents of the community. The Health Information Tool for Empowerment interactive website brings new resources to community-based organizations and institutions in matching community residents with needed services. The DentCare network brings dental facilities to public schools and, in the process of providing care, also educates children and teachers in the classroom about oral health issues.

Many of the pilot projects are being sustained by the groups that participated in planning and implementing them. For example, the School of Public Health and Alianza are continuing their work with educating community health workers, and the Ambulatory Care System of New York Presbyterian Hospital enjoys enhanced capacity to provide mental health care to the public.

On the policy front, mental health care now has parity with general health care: the Mental Health Parity bill was signed into law in 2008. A national organization for community health workers has been established to add their voices to improving the health care system for the poor in the United States.

There are many more examples of how the NMCVC improved the capacity of the community to educate itself and of sustained initiatives

begun by the NMCVC. From the outset the NMCVC did not envision creating a new entity or organization; rather, we wished to work through the
existing institutions and community-based organizations—and we have
been successful in reaching that goal.

So too can it be said that the institutions and the community worked together successfully. Since the lessons learned here are the ones that are important for future collaborations between universities and their academic
health centers and the community, we will explore in greater depth what we
learned about successful collaborations of this type. Overall we learned
that successful collaborations are built on two main principles: collaboration must be built on trusting relations, and a durable collaboration between universities, hospitals, and community-based organizations requires
a keen understanding of mission, mutual interests, and a willingness to re-
consider mission. Each of these findings is filled with many lessons.

Institutional–Community Collaboration: Building Trust

To say that building trust is neither simple nor easy would be an understatement. We discovered several interlocking components in operating
under this principle.

Understand the history. In building trusting relationships, we found it is
first necessary to understand the context and history of the institutions in
relation to their particular community. The NMCVC operated in two complex low-income communities of approximately 400,000 people: Washington Heights/Inwood, which is a largely Latino immigrant community
of which Dominicans are the greatest proportion; and Harlem, which is
mainly an African American community. Presbyterian Hospital, now New
York Presbyterian Hospital, and Columbia University Medical Center are
the dominant institutions in Washington Heights/Inwood—they are the
largest employers and also hold large blocks of real estate in the community. The main campus of Columbia University is only a stone's throw from
Harlem in Morningside Heights, where they are also the largest employers
and large real estate owners.

The relationships between these two northern Manhattan communities and the large institutions located in them had been strained over a
long period of time. Columbia, which sits on a hill, has had an uneasy
relationship with the Harlem community below and just east of it. So has

New York Presbyterian Hospital with the Latino population of Washington Heights/Inwood. Both institutions were viewed by their surrounding communities as elitist, and over a long period of time they clashed over a number of issues, continually reinforcing this opinion. For example, in Columbia's case, the well-known dispute about Columbia's plans to build a gymnasium in Morningside Park, the park that separates Columbia's campus from the Harlem community below it, sparked widespread community protests in the 1960s and still haunts relationships today. More recently, new strains with the community have developed over the expansion of the university campus into West Harlem (also known as Manhattanville).

Recognize the need to repair relationships. By the time the Community Voices program emerged in the late 1990s, however, both institutions had recognized the need to repair relationships with the community and had taken some steps to do so. The Columbia University Medical Center had appointed Ivy Fairchild as associate vice president for government and community affairs (see also chapter 13). As a Latina of Dominican heritage raised in the community, Fairchild was trusted by the community. She began outreach to community-based groups in northern Manhattan and was a strong supporter of the NMCVC. Fairchild recognized the importance from the community's perspective of the plans to construct the Thelma C. Davidson Adair Medical and Dental Center in a historic building in central Harlem and advocated for the center to be a university-wide endeavor.

The hospital administration also understood that it needed to improve relationships with the community surrounding it. New York Presbyterian Hospital (NYPH) is an internationally known hospital that has always served what is known as the "carriage trade" in New York City as well as high-profile individuals. For example, Bill Clinton had his bypass surgery done at the hospital. However, to get the approval of the New York State Health Department to construct a new facility in Washington Heights, a largely immigrant community, the NYPH was required to construct neighborhood primary care facilities in northern Manhattan and to build a community hospital north of its main location. NYPH was the last remaining hospital in northern Manhattan and had to serve both as a tertiary care hospital and a community hospital. To accomplish this dual role, the hospital administration recognized it was time to mend relationships with the community. They appointed Walid Michelen, who was a Latino of Dominican heritage, as medical director of the neighborhood ambulatory care facilities and the community hospital. Michelen became a key member of the NYPH staff and active participant of the NMCVC. He explained the climate in the community in the 1980s prior to building the new hospital facility: "The hospital wanted to build the Milstein Pavilion, an immense, modern structure for that time in order to compete for patients with commercial insurance. The community and others strongly protested the decision since they felt that the Medical Center had largely ignored the working class and underserved populations in its own backyard."

The community too wanted to develop better relationships with the institutions in northern Manhattan. Moisés Pérez, the executive director of the Alianza Dominicana (see chapter 3), says he "recognized that the NMCVC presented an opportunity to reconcile relationships and restore trust among the community and the big institutions, like Columbia." Thus, in developing a trusting relationship, one must first recognize the issues that have separated the parties and that have caused the strains. Both parties, in this case the large institutions in northern Manhattan and the community-based organizations that represented the residents, also must express a desire and a readiness to work together despite past differences.

Genuine interest in building relationships: Furthering trust depends too on whether the leadership placed in charge of a community-institutional collaborative program has a track record of accomplishments in projects recognized as genuinely sensitive to community concerns as well as having the respect of the institutions. The community needs to recognize that the relationship with the institutions cannot be one-sided and requires mutual self-interest. In the case of the NMCVC, the three partners (chapter 3) had that reputation. The dental school was a well-respected part of Columbia University. It had shown its concern for the community in the early 1990s by establishing the Community DentCare network, a public school- and neighborhood-based system of oral health care. The Harlem Hospital Dental Service had collaborated extensively with the dental school, and the university was eager to improve the affiliation with the hospital (see also the epilogue). The Harlem Hospital Dental Service expanded its services in the 1980s beyond mainly an acute care program of extractions to provide comprehensive dental care; this was much appreciated by the community. Alianza had been working with youth and families and with public and private institutions to improve distressed neighborhoods since 1987. Because the university and the hospital were anxious to improve their relationship with the community, both supported the goals of the NMCVC. That the three partners that came together to plan and establish the

NMCVC had previous working relations and understood their respective environments was another advantage.

Relationships become especially important for the major research universities when dealing with their communities. A community member expressed one of the biggest complaints in university–community relationships when she said, "We no longer want to be research subjects for someone's funded research project. We have too often been left with nothing after cooperating with a researcher's project. What we want are service programs, programs that can deal with uplifting the community. We understand that such service projects may have a research and education component, but we do not any longer wish to be simply studied. We also want to be at the table in planning community-based initiatives." The Community DentCare project followed that new model of cooperation. It was a service model that had both education and research components as secondary to the service mission. The NMCVC was launched with great promise to be an effective way to bring all partners to the table. It was important that trust continued to be built in all parameters of the collaborative.

Work at the grass roots. It was important to put into place a structure that would further build trusting relations and then to place individuals who had the ability to communicate with both the institutions and the community in critical positions. In developing the structure and the processes that the NMCVC used to interact with the institutions and the community, the actual work of the NMCVC happened at the grass-roots level in the working groups. The leadership of these groups was composed of individuals who gained the confidence of the community-based organizations they engaged as well as the hospital and the university. In the various chapters examples abound of the ways in which the leadership went about reinforcing trust. A few examples illustrate this point.

- Findley and Michelen (chapter 3), the cochairs of the Health Promotion/Disease Prevention working group, held numerous meetings with community groups and surveyed the community on their perceptions of the problems affecting the communities' health. They interviewed 482 community residents, 48 providers, and the leaders of 11 community-based organizations.
- Instead of jumping headlong into the mental health issues, Hernández-Cordero (chapter 12) worked to understand the factors

affecting the providers of mental health care and the communities'
perspectives of the problem. A series of interviews with community-
based agencies and health care institutions was matched by discussion groups with both consumers and nonconsumers of mental
health services. The Mental Health Report that came from this effort
has been used extensively over the last decade and still serves today
as a framework for improving the mental health safety net in northern Manhattan.

• The widespread use of community health workers in the
NMCVC (see particularly chapter 3) built trust with community residents. Individuals who previously would not sign up for Medicaid
because they were concerned about government misuse of their personal information decided to enroll. In fact, thirty thousand children
and adults came into the program when community health workers
whom they trusted were the agents to sign them up. In every NMCVC
initiative that depended upon a trusting relationship between provider and community resident, community health workers became
the bridge to success. They were incorporated into the asthma and
the immunization projects (chapters 4 and 5), into the tobacco cessation initiatives (chapter 6), and into SASA (chapter 7).

Ability to play to a dual audience. It was not enough for the working
group leaders to develop the trust of the community. They also had to have
credibility and active participation of key stakeholders within the major
institutions involved in the partnership. Playing to this dual audience was
not easy and required individuals of great sensitivity. All of the university
faculty who participated in the NMCVC were respected members of their
faculties. For example:

• Findley, a clinical professor, had the confidence of the dean of
the School of Public Health and her department head.
• Marshall was able to bring together the necessary resources to
build the DentCare network because he had been shown to be an
able administrator and a good manager.
• Seidman was a knowledgeable researcher in tobacco and developed good working relationships in the dental school, enabling him
to build the tobacco cessation clinic there.

- While initially the hospital was reluctant to participate in the NMCVC, it was convinced to do so by Michelen, the individual it hired to help the hospital's outreach to the community.
- The Thelma C. Davidson Adair Medical and Dental Center in Harlem was supported by the university and Medical Center because the then president of the university (George Rupp) and interim dean of the medical school (Thomas Morris) had trust in Formicola as the longtime dean of the dental school. Morris and Formicola also co-chaired one of the four NMCVC working groups.

In addition, the first two executive directors of NMCVC, Sandra Harris and Jacqueline Martínez, and the program coordinator, Yisel Alonzo, were from the community. They had grown up in northern Manhattan and had gone on to higher education but had not forgotten their roots. While Lourdes Hernández-Cordero had not grown up in the community, she put down roots there by living and raising her family in its heart. All four of the critical staff members understood the culture of the communities, respected the opinions of their representatives, and had the ability to communicate with everyone—from heads of community-based organizations to clergy, and from elected members of New York City government to state officials. Their credibility became the face of the NMCVC. It became apparent that the executive leadership of the NMCVC was able to show to the community that the university and hospitals were willing to address concerns of importance to the community. It was fortunate that each of these leaders originally came from the community or lived in it and had advanced their education in public health and in health education at the masters and doctoral levels. They were well grounded in community issues and became trusted members of the institutions.

From our vantage point, we learned that relationships are primary, just as we had been told in our first annual meeting with all thirteen Community Voices sites. And, while that seems intuitive, when we sat down to develop the NMCVC we did not explicitly set down this principle as a founding principle of the collaborative. It just worked out that way. We were fortunate to bring forth the right combination of people. As described in chapter 2, we put "onto the bus" those who had the ability to take the initial desire of the institutions and the community to come together and build it into a cooperative endeavor. We set up systems that continually regenerated and enabled these kinds of leaders. In summing up, this emerges as the first principle of a successful collaborative: trust is an imperative for success.

Harmony Among Mission, Goals, and Financial Feasibility

The second important principle that emerged from the NMCVC learning laboratory is that there is a need for fit between initiatives and the mission, goals, and feasibility of the host institutions and community organizations to institutionalize initiatives. This could be called staying within the comfort zone of the established institutions and community-based organizations. We learned that for an initiative to take hold and sustain itself from pilot project to mature program, it had to intersect with the mission, goals, and financial interests/abilities of the institutions and organizations within the community. Just as important, a project also had to be part of the culture of the community.

The Asthma Basics for Children (ABC) program (chapter 4) is an example of a successful relationship between a program and the partners' mission and goals. Each of the participating partners took on responsibilities for the parts of the program that best fit their mission and core strengths. The Mailman School of Public Health was responsible for evaluation, reporting, and fund raising. Two community groups, the Northern Manhattan Improvement Corporation in Washington Heights and the Northern Manhattan Perinatal Partnership in Harlem, took on the management and oversight for all of the participating ABC community programs. Altogether there were fifty-six different participating programs. Wisely, the leadership of the ABC program understood that the mission of the participating programs included education and integrated the ABC program into the work of the existing programs rather than start a stand-alone program. Findley and Michelen knew that the program needed to rest on the principle of "by the community, for the community" and placed the action at the community level, which was in tune with what the community groups do, and reserved for the School of Public Health those elements that were well within the scope of its mission.

Another example of harmony between mission and program is the facilitated enrollment program for eligible individuals into Medicaid and Child Health Plus insurance. Alianza Dominicana viewed it as within its core mission to help the community get resources that would improve their lives. Therefore, helping people become enrolled in health insurance was well within its mission. Similarly, Alianza partnered with the Mailman School of Public Health to develop a certificate program for educating community health workers because education is within the mission of the university. Specifically, the School of Public Health understood that creating a community health worker educational track related to the important work of creating a new worker who could intervene at the community level. The School of Public Health and Alianza, working within their respective missions, were responsible for community health workers becoming the bedrock of most of the initiatives undertaken in northern Manhattan.

When projects were not within the well-understood mission, they were not sustainable. Healthy Choices and the Thelma C. Davidson Adair Medical and Dental Center are examples of two projects that fit into this category. The Healthy Choices program ran a successful pilot test to address obesity in the community, but it depended on using the public school system as the setting for the program (chapter 10). Given the myriad of issues the public school system was facing, the superintendent of schools, who was a supporter of the program, was unable to adopt the program system-wide. Educating parents on proper diet, nutrition, and exercise was not within the core mission of the public school system, so while the pilot test had a successful outcome, the program was not adopted in the public school system. This initiative was clearly out of the boundaries of the mission of those that would have to adopt it and sustain it over time.

The Thelma C. Davidson Adair Medical and Dental Center is a much more complex situation that mixes a lack of harmony between perceived mission and financial viability (see chapter 13). From the community perspective, the center located in Central Harlem was a vanguard of better times for the community and improved relationships between Harlem and Columbia University. A health facility built on the philosophy of a Park Avenue practice with scheduled appointments rather than another clinic where patients wait all day to see a provider was a harbinger of the growing upgrading of the Harlem community. Through the opening of the center, there was good will generated for the university during a time of stormy relations with the community because of the university's expansion plans into West Harlem. But ultimately, the university and the medical and dental schools did not wish to continue to operate the center.

What went wrong? There were two major reasons why the university and the medical and dental schools did not wish to continue operating the center: finances and perceived ill fit into the mission. On the one hand, the medical and dental schools were simply not prepared to subsidize long term a freestanding primary care health center in Harlem. The center had accumulated a $1 million debt with the university for operating start-up costs and an operating deficit in the range of approximately $80,000 to $100,000 per year in the last two of its six years of operating under the umbrella of the university. Primary care centers in New York were all having financial problems, and the Adair Center was not an exception. But most primary care centers are operated by Federally Qualified Health Centers or community health centers and/or hospitals that could find other ways to subsidize their operating deficits for these primary care facilities. Most of the parent organizations of primary care centers are owned by entities that support the facilities as key to their main mission.

On the other hand, the university's main mission is research and education. Thus, although the medical and dental schools view patient care as a mission, the medical school uses a separate entity (the hospital or incorporated faculty practices) as the setting for its patient care mission; the dental school operates on-site teaching clinics, which can be cross-subsidized because they are teaching clinics. The Adair Center most likely could have closed the gap on its operating deficit and paid back the university loan, but it would have taken several more years for that to happen. With the center's unresolved financial issues and little to do with the main mission (education and research) in the eyes of the leadership within the medical and dental schools, the university's will to sustain it was just not there.

There is another side to this story that brings out a further important point about mission: mission can be interpreted differently by different leaders. A previous leadership team who developed the Adair Center did see the center within the mission, or were willing to stretch the mission, because they believed it was in the enlightened self-interest of the university and the health science schools. Their view was that the annual amount that needed to be subsidized could have been raised, and that the center had the capacity to provide opportunities to undertake education of students and residents and research potential as it provided services to the community. However, with a change of leadership at the school and university levels, there was a lack of willingness to continue sponsoring the Adair Center.

With a change in leadership, there were also conflicting viewpoints about the center's importance to the building of good relationships between the university and the Harlem community and its importance to the core mission of education and research. Whether these same conflicts would have come about if this had not occurred during a time of great financial stress for the university and the medical school, which was under great pressure to balance its budget, can only be speculated about. What is clear, however, is that in the eyes of Thelma Adair, this was a sad commentary on the university's willingness to be a good citizen of the community. Upon learning of the university's plans to close the center, this icon of the Harlem community observed that "after finally coming down from the Hill to work with the people of Harlem," Columbia University lost an opportunity by closing the center located in an historic Harlem building. The fact that the university could not sustain the center shows that when a program is conceived of as peripheral to the mission by its leaders (or the leaders are not able to view the mission more broadly as in the self-interest of the institution) and is not a winner financially, it does not gain the internal support needed for it to succeed long term.

The leaders who planned and pushed for the Adair Center were mistaken in thinking that a primary care center could be housed in the university, at least in Columbia University. Despite the painful lessons learned in the Adair Center story, we have a happy ending. The center has been taken over by a well-respected Federally Qualified Health Center, the Ryan Center. And, the medical and dental schools generously agreed to turn over the $2.6 million center to Ryan at no cost. The current $1 million debt owed to the university will not be passed onto Ryan. We could have simply called the project a success given that a fine facility will continue to be available to the community, hence improving the safety net for the community. However, as learning laboratories it is important for us to bring out the lessons learned in order to help others who aspire to work in collaborations between community and institutions.

Summary of Lessons Learned

The lessons learned through the NMCVC are not simply a list of all the things that went well. Rather, as in any iterative process, they synthesize the successes, failures, and challenges faced and how we went about incorporating each into adapting our original plan. In summary, lessons learned are:

1. Trusting relationships are primary. The NMCVC was built on the good will between the original partners and operated to build trust with all of its collaborators. Cultural awareness and individuals that can deliver are essential to success.

2. Initiatives need to fit harmoniously into the missions, goals, and needs of institutions and the communities. Reward systems of the organization or institution help to maintain staff and faculty interests and to secure a place within the organization or institution for the program.

3. Collaborations between universities and health science centers and their communities can plan and implement highly successful programs to improve the health of the community. The leadership on both sides for such efforts—the institutions and the community-based organizations—need to understand that the mutual self-interest of each must be respected. The institutions, usually large employers and real estate holders in the community, must be willing to extend themselves to create a positive working climate with their respective communities.

Finally, the Community Voices initiative of the W. K. Kellogg Foundation demonstrated that the nation's largest foundations have a major impact on important social issues confronting our country and those who participate in one of their grant programs. In the first five years, the NMCVC was awarded a $4.5 million grant. The grant funds were awarded to the dental school, which then provided funds to the various initiatives. Major funds were provided to Alianza Dominicana and Community Premier Plus. The School of Public Health received funds for support of faculty and student scholars, as did the dental and medical schools. Funding to a variety of community-based organizations helped ensure that their efforts were supported financially. The initiative also leveraged additional funds from other foundations and state and federal sources. These additional funds were considerable, amounting to over $45 million.

During this first five years, then, funding was partially responsible for bringing the partnership together and helped keep it together. The steering committee met regularly, as did the working groups. However, it was never the perception of the partners that the funding is what brought people to the table—although we are sure there were some people who did feel that it was the funding that kept them there. It is not a perfect world, and leadership needs to recognize this fact.

It was the interesting, unique, and exciting opportunity to work across traditional institutional and community boundaries that mainly kept people together. Being part of a national program brought a sense of pride to both the community and the institutional partners that allowed us to bring people together in the first five years of the program. During the last four years, we had a grant of $1 million to spend on developing policy initiatives to sustain projects begun in the first phase. This required the collaborative to move from working with local groups to state and national groups. In this phase, the NMCVC concentrated on policy to recognize community health workers as health care workers so that they could be compensated by insurance companies and Medicaid/Medicare funds and to advocate for obtaining parity between funding for mental health and for other health care services. While the NMCVC was successful in helping both of these policy initiatives to come about, interest in the NMCVC by the large group of collaborators waned after the first five years. Most likely the shift to policy—a more abstract endeavor and harder to link to work on the ground—was responsible for the loss of interest by most of the groups with which we worked. We probably missed a great opportunity in not celebrating the successes of the NMCVC as we moved from one phase of the work to another and perhaps lost the "brand name" we had developed at the community level.

There is not a good way to wind down an initiative such as this one. We kept working on initiatives during the last four years, such as the Adair Center, HITE, and the Healthy Choices program, because the staff was committed to improving the community. On balance, the NMCVC was able to create a positive climate for a ten-year period of cooperation between numerous community-based organizations and institutions. It was the people who came together that made the project a success. Many of them went on to successful new endeavors as a result of participating in the NMCVC. In the epilogue we tell some of the other stories of how partners continue the work after the NMCVC.

Thus far this book has chronicled the effort and has attempted to put it into perspective as the nation grapples with ways to improve the health of its citizens. In the final chapter we discuss approaches to scale up some of the lessons learned to the national health care reform movement now going on in the country.

References

Columbia's west Harlem expansion: A look at the issues. http://www.columbia.edu/cu/cssn/expansion/. . . /scegbooklet(short-edge).pdf.

Columbia University planning program website. http://neighbors.columbia.edu/pages/manplanning/.

Morningside Heights website. http://www.morningside-heights.net/gym.htm.

Scaling Up

LOURDES HERNÁNDEZ-CORDERO, SUSAN STURM,
KATHLEEN KLINK, and ALLAN J. FORMICOLA

When I chose to be a public health practitioner I did so because I had the need to be of service to others. I had always focused on what I, as an individual, could do to improve the life of the collective— of my neighborhood, my workplace, and my "target community." I have never spoken about how the principles that guide my work could improve the health of the nation. I always thought that an individual voice was necessary but that it took community voices to make a change at a bigger scale.

—Lourdes Hernández-Cordero

Moments of crisis require big, bold ideas. In this chapter we will zoom out of our close examination of the Northern Manhattan Community Voices Collaborative experience to propose ways to scale up the things that worked for us in order to make them applicable at a national level. With this chapter we honor the intent of the W. K. Kellogg Foundation in its support of learning laboratories across the nation. Our goal is to contribute to the collective dialogue on how to improve the health care system. Specifically, we propose that making a healthier nation and reducing health care costs will require more than simply moving toward universal health coverage— which is essential—or implementing technologies to digitalize medical records—which is useful. As epidemiologists would say, those things are necessary but not sufficient to overhaul our ailing health care system. Instead, we propose to reduce health care costs and improve health care access by implementing a national prevention program through collaboration based on a new health compact with society—one that delivers on the promise of justice for all and (paraphrasing our forefathers/mothers) the pursuit of health.

In the previous chapter we summed up the ten-year experience of NMCVC. In this chapter we propose building on that experience and thinking broadly to solve the problems of our health care system. We will begin by defining and making the case for prevention as the cornerstone of a new health care system. Second, we will make the connection between prevention and collaboration and will draw on the Community Voices experience to propose a large-scale movement toward prevention through collaboration that activates the network of academic and community health centers and their respective community partners. Finally, we will outline a blueprint for the implementation of these ideas and provide examples of the types of policies that could make the blueprint a reality.

Here's to being bold.

Making the Case for Prevention

The nation is once more engaged in an exercise to reform our health care system. At the heart of this new round is a debate about whether and how to cover all Americans and how to improve the quality of care. We believe that this debate misses the mark if it does not address how the role of prevention can become a pillar of health reform. We also believe that the government acting alone will not be able to provide greater access to health care services and foster the systemic changes needed to improve quality of care. This task will require the involvement of many other stakeholders, including academic and community health centers, public health practitioners, and grassroots community organizers. Furthermore, since the new reality of the health status of the American people is that chronic illness constitutes the biggest burden, a system that was largely planned to contain acute illness is inadequate. Therefore, the health care system needs to be not only restructured but also reconceptualized. A reconceptualized health care system that puts prevention, promotion of healthy behaviors, and management of chronic illness at the heart of the new plan will benefit not only underserved population groups living in inner cities and rural areas that are marginalized in regard to health, but also the average American who sometimes perceives the burden of the *cost* of health care to fall on her or his shoulders.

> BOX 15.1
>
> *Defining Prevention*
>
> We define prevention as activities that fall within three categories: preventive medical care, wellness promotion, and chronic disease management.
>
> *Preventive medical care*: Clinical interventions including examinations, screenings, measures that guard against disease, injury avoidance driven by risk assessments, and standardized protocols. Aimed at avoiding the onset of illness and early detection.
>
> *Wellness promotion*: Education and facilitation leading to healthy behaviors related to physical activity, nutritious eating, sun safety, alcohol, tobacco and other drug use, and violence prevention. Education is aimed at acquiring knowledge, shaping attitudes, and developing competency. Facilitation is aimed at improving access to healthy options and creating safe and just environments.
>
> *Chronic disease management*: Treatment and close monitoring of chronic illnesses once they have been diagnosed.

Prevention as the Cornerstone of a New Health Care System

A lot has been said about what prevention can or cannot do. The jury is still out in many ways with regard to how much (or if) prevention can help reduce health care costs. Some preventive measures that are highly valuable (e.g., flu shots, cervical and prostate cancer screenings, cholesterol and high blood pressure screenings) are not necessarily cost-savers. Other preventive measures (e.g., vaccinations for toddlers, vision and hearing screenings), wellness promotion, and chronic illness management strategies have mountains of evidence supporting their cost-saving benefits.

TABLE 15.1

The Economics of Prevention

Net savings in health care costs of an investment of $10 per person per year in
  proven community-based disease prevention programs:
In 1–2 years: $2.8 billion annually
Within 5 years: $16 billion annually
Within 10–20 years: $18 billion annually

Source: Trust for America's Health (2008).

A New Health Compact

However, there are more important reasons for putting prevention at the
center of a health care system than cost savings. Putting prevention as the
cornerstone of the health care system is the right thing to do. The great
health compacts that gave us Medicare and Medicaid raised our expectations that—just as education is seen as a right—access to basic health care
would also be a right. Now, almost forty-five years later, our nation has
veered from this direction in benefit of economic interests and has bought
into the idea that health care benefits are a privilege. Bold, swift action is
required to call to task a variety of stakeholders—from academia to service
providers, from professionals to lay health workers. Bold, swift action is
needed to make activities serve more than one purpose—to rethink service as a way to learn, and as a way to serve. Bold, swift action is indispens-
able to regain a leading role globally as a just and fair country that cares for
its citizens—all of them, not just the ones who can afford it. Bold, swift
action is needed to change the status quo.

There are two main reasons why fostering prevention is the right thing
to do: equality and opportunity. Prevention is about equality because the
bulk of the burden of disease and illness falls on the poor and people of
color. Reducing their share of the burden would be a step toward reducing
health disparities. Prevention is also about opportunity because there is a
close link between health status and economic attainment. The direction
of the relationship between health and education or health and economic
status is not clear yet. That is, we do not know with certainty if people who are
sick do less well in school because of their illness *or* if being more educated
can inform and enable people to choose healthy behaviors. The research

evidence, however, indicates that there is a direct correlation between health and level of education as well as health and socioeconomic status. That is, the higher a person's level of education, the better their general health. The higher their socioeconomic status (i.e., earning a living wage, having stable housing), the better their general health.

Coverage for everyone is one way of improving the health care system. But it is not the only way. We propose that an important step toward improving the health care system is to enact a new health compact that flips the current system toward prevention as the priority.

Prevention Through Collaboration

The connection between prevention and collaboration is not obvious at first. If, after reading this chapter, it becomes apparent and logical, we would have fulfilled our goal to contribute to the collective dialogue on how to improve the health care system and sowed the seeds of making prevention a national priority.

The tasks we call for to make prevention a cornerstone of the national health care system—preventive medical care, wellness promotion, and chronic disease management—are not difficult to understand. They are, however, complex to achieve. The reason why they are complex is that they require not only the kind of knowledge generated through research (e.g., the discoveries of new and effective treatment options, the identification of risk and protective factors that can be altered through healthy behaviors, standardized protocols), but also knowledge about translating research into practice, about adapting strategies to make them culturally relevant, and about the "goodness of fit" of an initiative to local needs and resources. Some of this knowledge is contained outside of the institutions that are part of the health care system, and within the community itself.

We propose that prevention works best when many stakeholders are involved in the planning, dissemination, and implementation of activities because each stakeholder brings a unique and crucial perspective. Going from a one-dimensional view of a problem to a multidimensional view compensates for any organizational blind spots that may exist. Collaboration is the mechanism through which stakeholders can be convened and work can be carried out.

The Community Voices Experience

Reviewing the work of the NMCVC, three lessons for effective collaboration can be distilled: (1) community–institutional collaboration can lead
to successful community-wide prevention initiatives; (2) prevention initiatives can be put into place when set within the mission of an institution
and partnering organizations (a corollary of this lesson is that sometimes
outside "carrots and sticks" must be used to restate the mission of an institution to be in line with the goals of the prevention tasks); and (3) cooperation between institutions and community-based organizations in underserved urban areas can lead to increased capacity for prevention, a richer
learning environment grounded in service, and opportunities for cutting-
edge research that benefits all stakeholders.

A Large-Scale Movement Toward Prevention

The proposal we make is ambitious and only possible if an equally ambitious challenge is posed to the stakeholders we aim to mobilize. The challenge we propose is that all academic and health centers expand their missions to put service as an important component of what they do rather
than a byproduct of afterthought of their intellectual and clinical pursuits.
Service provides the way to connect teaching and research. When treated as
a core activity, it offers a way to develop a research agenda with the promise
of improving the health status of underserved communities. When treated
as a way to equip students to advance a public health mission, service en-
nobles teaching and enables learning. When you think of service as an
opportunity for learning, it naturally becomes part of a curriculum that
prepares professionals for real life. When you think of service as an important application of intellectual work, it can lead to cutting-edge research
that benefits both the researchers and research participants. Service is a
valid way to build a professional record of excellence while also building
the trust of the communities in which one works.

Public health and health science professionals from all over the nation
affiliated with institutions that share a backyard with impoverished communities can provide service that advances the prevention agenda while
also meeting the goals of their funders and receiving accolades for their

scientifically rigorous work. For this to happen, a shift in institutional mission and what is valued must occur to include addressing health care needs of underserved communities. And this shift can be accomplished by strategically linking funding and reporting priorities to a service component, successfully activating a vast network of academic and health centers.

Activating Academic and Health Centers and Their Community Partners

The idea of community–university partnerships is not new. The U.S. Department of Housing and Urban Development has an Office of University Partnerships that funds and supports campus–community partnerships aimed at economic development through job creation and neighborhood building. Similarly the Community–Campus Partnerships for Health, a nonprofit organization, facilitates partnerships between communities and institutions of higher education aimed at promoting health.

The NMCVC brought together several schools from the Columbia University Medical Center. The Medical Center is home to a dental school, a medical school, a public health school, a nursing school, and a nutrition institute. While only three of those institutions were actively involved in the first nine years of the project, the renamed Center for Family and Community Medicine has sought to engage also the nursing and nutrition faculty. The kind of mobilization for prevention that we propose would activate the vast network of academic and health centers across the nation to collaborate with community-based organizations in their own backyard by linking incentives (funding, recognition, accreditation credit) and creating policies to ensure that prevention activities are a priority in the work, service, and research agenda of academic and health centers.

Think about the potential for national reach.

There are 158 accredited medical schools, 40 accredited schools of public health, 58 accredited dental schools, and 468 nursing schools and programs. This list includes private and public institutions, big and small, based in urban and rural areas. Furthermore, there are 1,067 Federally Qualified Health Centers and over 7,000 community health centers throughout all fifty states and the U.S. territories.

Now imagine the possibilities.

Blueprint for Collaboration

We propose a plan to meet the health needs of all Americans that is based on the principles of (1) a national health care system that prioritizes prevention and (2) policies that reward and foster collaboration. Prioritizing prevention means flipping the health care system's priorities from a crisis-reaction-driven system that reveres specialization to a proactive system grounded in primary care and collective solutions. We believe that by expanding what we consider to be the purview of the health care system beyond the medical encounter, we can reach so many more people—especially the underserved who carry a disproportionate burden of disease—and so begin to "mind" the health gap. Fostering collaboration for prevention is the framework for success. The policies and incentives we call for would help identify a broader set of stakeholders, a more comprehensive set of priorities, and a series of mechanisms that build on research and learning/teaching to increase and improve service. Mechanisms for research and learning/teaching that encourage real-life, community-based collaborations need not sacrifice scientific integrity or academic freedom. On the contrary, we propose that these new mechanisms encourage creative problem solving, research in in vivo settings that can be translatable, and a rich learning environment that at the same time provides much needed service. Research for the sake of research is not good enough. Service without a research or evaluation component is not good enough either. These two tasks must complement each other. When they do, teaching and learning are enhanced. Next, we present the who, how, and what of the blueprint for collaboration.

Who: Broad Array of Stakeholders

We propose that the "who"—the stakeholders—carrying out collaboration for prevention should include academic health centers, community health centers, advocacy groups, public bodies, intermediaries, and foundations. All of the stakeholders may not be present in every community, nor may they be the right partners for all initiatives undertaken. Nonetheless, they all need to be engaged for a nationwide mobilization to occur.

Academic health centers have the responsibility to train health care professionals and the opportunity to provide services through the training experience. For example, practica, internships, and faculty who provide care or technical assistance while teaching are all resources that academic health centers can bring to collaborations. All of these activities can become part of the research portfolio (i.e., as evaluations, Community-Based Participatory Action Research, or translational research). Through the NMCVC years, we learned about leveraging the role of academic health centers as anchor institutions for collaboration. They are in a position to develop the new generation of transformative leaders committed to ongoing collaboration and knowledge development. As recipients of tax exemptions and indirect costs from government grants, academic health centers have accepted public support for their work. Therefore, policy could and should be deployed to encourage these institutions to promote responsibility for community health as part of their core mission by requiring active collaboration with community-based organizations with which they would interact in assessing priorities, designing programs, and managing the ongoing process of helping develop the national health system.

Community health centers—many located in medical shortage areas—are also anchor institutions and an important venue for the deployment of information, program implementation, and convening of stakeholders. Collaboration would boost a community health center's ability to carry out prevention activities, to serve as a site for wellness promotion, and to effectively manage chronic illness. As the flagship institutions for primary care delivery, community health centers are a keystone in flipping the health care system toward prevention.

Advocacy groups, which are mainly community-based organizations, are essential not only because they serve as the "voices" of the community, but also as drivers of policy that is informed by reality. Because of their intimate knowledge of communities and the populations that they serve (and represent), they are a vital sounding board in policy development and enactment as well as the logical leaders in many prevention activities.

Public bodies (in the case of northern Manhattan, the City Council and the Community Boards) in many instances have a bird's-eye view of what is going on programmatically in the community. When public bodies are incorporated as collaborators, duplication of efforts is minimized and synergy can be garnered.

Intermediaries are boundary-spanning institutions that operate across multiple systems, organizations, and fields. Community Voices became this kind of cross-cutting catalyst that brought together different groups to address shared problems and mobilize change. These intermediaries play a crucial role in creating space for ongoing collaboration and maintaining linkages across the silos that typically separate universities, communities, and policy makers. They also translate the needs and insights of these groups to policy makers and funders.

Foundations can be key intermediaries providing an architecture to support ongoing change. The W. K. Kellogg Foundation's role as the catalyst for Community Voices offers one example of how an intermediary can use resources to stimulate a process of leadership, collaboration, reflection, problem solving, and institutional change that makes good business sense. In our story, foundations featured prominently as agents that allowed us to solidify, legitimize, and elevate the impact of our work.

How: A Multilevel Ecological Approach

One of the most striking things about the Community Voices story is the number of people from different positions and backgrounds who worked together to bring about change over a long period of time. This kind of multilevel, long-term collaboration was crucial to the successful adoption of prevention as a strategy. The Community Voices story illustrates how a multilevel, ecological approach can take hold by creating an architecture supporting ongoing learning, transformative leadership, long-term university–community partnerships, and systems change. A convergence of commitment among leaders within the community, the university, health care institutions, and foundations gave rise to an infrastructure to support ongoing change. We propose that by taking an ecological approach, the role of all stakeholders in the overall design of the health care system could be sustained and could provide the driving force for prevention through collaboration.

What: Building Collaborations for Prevention

We are proposing a large-scale initiative aimed at making a healthier nation. The initiative will reduce health care costs through collaboration for prevention. Flipping the current health care system to prioritize prevention is, admittedly, a huge undertaking. Fortunately, there is no need to start from scratch. Drawing on the local experience of the NMCVC, we believe the following blueprint can form the basis for a mobilization effort on a national scale.

Enlist organizational leaders. Within organizations, visionary leaders with fresh thinking and an understanding of the benefits of a health care system grounded on prevention should be identified. These leaders will bring core institutional support to the collaboration and ensure long-term support for joint activities. Educational and health policy should foster the development of new leaders with vision, commitment, and organizational ability.

Pay attention to structure. While the NMCVC counted over thirty-five partner organizations, not all participated in every initiative. A structure was set in place (working groups, executive and steering committees) that enabled participants to get things done, to gather data needed to inform action, and to learn from those who had the knowledge of what was needed and what would work. The partners involved in each specific initiative varied according to their expertise, interests, and capacity.

Keep relationships first. Requests for proposals may come and go, but relationships will remain. Relationships are built on small gestures (e.g., attending an event or meeting for the sake of support, even if no immediate benefit is secured) and support big efforts (e.g., large-scale projects, sharing of resources).

Articulate a joint, affirmative vision. State what stakeholders stand for (instead of what they are against) and how they want to go about achieving a community-wide goal of health for all. This vision then becomes the rule of thumb measured against all new projects. If a new initiative does not pass muster, then it is a diversion and the collaborative is better off passing on it than losing its focus.

Seek mutuality, practice reciprocity. Look for those things in common that stakeholders may have. They may not all agree on all issues, but a working agenda can be drafted based on common goals. Once commonalities are found, strive to exchange resources, services, favors, or obligations. A collaboration can be built this way in the absence of (or while waiting for) external funding.

Map and match like things. List and map all existing policies or activities in the ecological framework articulated for the community at hand. This will aid stakeholders to match those initiatives or opportunities for easy wins—existing resources that can be shared, programming that can be enhanced, or information that can be disseminated.

Build capacity and infrastructure for ongoing organizational transforma-tion. By focusing on building capacity and infrastructure change, prevention can become second nature, the default position rather than a special activity or a deviation from the norm.

Develop organizational catalysts. Also referred to as "champions of a cause," leaders who are also catalysts understand that leading is more than managing. Good leadership enables the growth of all staff, the enhancement of programming, and the optimization of resources. In this regard, training community individuals, such as community health workers, as integral to prevention programs serves as a bridge between large institutions and community residents.

Sustain community participation and accountability. Design policies and programming with the goal of sustaining work beyond the funding period. Make all stakeholders accountable for their share and for providing checks and balances to others in an empowering way (rather than in a policing way).

Policies to Implement the Blueprint

For this blueprint to be implemented at the national level, we suggest the following list of policies (this not an exhaustive list):

- Prioritize public and private funding for prevention.
- Prioritize funding for research and training activities with an explicit service component.
- Implement incentives to promote collaboration.
- Favor long-standing collaborations, and foster new ones.
- Require systems for reflection and assessment in all funded projects. Reflectivity seeks a reality check, and evaluations seek to measure impact or change. Both are important and should be required as part of regular reporting and as a way to provide feedback to improve policies and initiatives.
- Connect individual innovation and systemic change. Create processes whereby experiences at the local level can be leveraged and inform the crafting of the new national health care system.

In summary, just as the participants in the Northern Manhattan Community Voices Collaborative sought to learn from and share their own experiences and struggles, this book is an effort to enhance the work of researchers, educators, and practitioners who also seek to engage in these efforts. Rather than a final word, it is the continuation of a dialogue.

References

Blane, D. (1995). Social determinants of health—socioeconomic status, social class, and ethnicity. *American Journal of Public Health* 85, no. 7: 903–5.

Centers for Disease Control and Prevention website. http://www.cdc.gov/NCCD PHP/tracking.htm.

Cohen, J. T., P. J. Neumann, and M. C. Weinstein (2008). Does preventive care save money? Health economics and the presidential candidates. *New England Journal of Medicine* 358, no. 26: 2847.

Community-Campus Partnerships for Health website. http://www.ccph.info.

Institute of Medicine (2004). *The future of the public's health in the 21st century. Committee on Assuring the Health of the Public in the 21st Century.* Washington, D.C.: National Academies Press.

Link, Bruce G., and Jo Phelan (1995). Social conditions as fundamental causes of disease. *Journal of Health and Social Behavior* 35 (Extra Issue): 80–94.

Office of University Partnerships website. http://www.oup.org.

Sturm, S. (2006). The architecture of inclusion: Advancing workplace equality in higher education. *Harvard Journal of Law and Gender* 29: 247–334.

—— (2007). Gender equity as institutional transformation: The pivotal role of "organizational catalysts." In *Transforming science and engineering: Advancing academic women*, ed. A. J. Stewart, J. E. Malley, and D. Lavaque-Manty, 260–80. Ann Arbor: University of Michigan Press.

U.S. Department of Health and Human Services. (1992). *Public Health Service. Healthy people 2000, Public Health Service action.* Washington, D.C.: U.S. Government Printing Office.

—— (2000). *Healthy people 2010: Understanding and improving health.* 2nd ed. Washington, D.C.: U.S. Government Printing Office.

U.S. Department of Health, Education and Welfare. (1979). *The surgeon general's report on health promotion and disease prevention.* Publication no. 79-55071. Washington, D.C.: U.S. Government Printing Office.

Epilogue

In this book we described the Northern Manhattan Community Voices Collaborative, how it came about, and the various projects it undertook. We discussed the outcomes of the ten-year initiative, which was one of the thirteen funded projects under the W. K. Kellogg Foundation's Community Voices: Health Care for the Underserved program. The three original partners, the Columbia University College of Dental Medicine, the Harlem Hospital Dental Service, and Alianza Dominicana, came together and built an organizational structure that served as a catalyst for improving the health care system for northern Manhattan residents. There were over thirty-five community-based organizations that in one way or another came together with the lead partners and several institutional partners, such as the Mailman School of Public Health, New York Presbyterian Hospital and the Greater New York Hospital Association. The collaborators were able to parlay a $4.5 million grant into over $45 million worth of subsequent efforts benefiting community health. In so doing, they strengthened community-wide prevention efforts and access to general and oral health care and enhanced the capacity of the community and the institutions to collaborate on issues of mutual concern.

To put this massive effort into perspective as to why the idea of Community Voices "stuck," we can look to the book *Made to Stick*. The authors,

Dan and Chip Heath, describe six principles on why some ideas are successful and stick. The principles for successful ideas that catch on are "Simple, Unexpected, Concrete, Credible, (and they evoke) Emotions and (engaging) Stories." We believe that the NMCVC had elements of all of these principles, and that the idea of prevention through collaboration we proposed in the chapter 15 will stick.

We think the ideas we presented in this book will catch the imagination of leadership in government, academic health institutions, the public health community, and the medical fields. It seems simple. We can make a healthier nation and reduce the costs of health care by implementing a national prevention program through collaboration. We presented concrete ways that the NMCVC actually accomplished this as examples for others. Community health workers are the credible agents of changing the behavior and the perceptions of residents to permit prevention to take hold across communities in need. We told several stories in the book that brought out feelings of trustworthiness and emphasized the emotional dimensions of community work. The idea of Community Voices has stuck in northern Manhattan.

It is also apparent that the three partners who created the NMCVC have stuck to their vision of community service and have continued to make other advances through collaboration. A few examples will demonstrate how the Community Voices principles live on. Alianza Dominicana has flourished as an important resource for the northern Manhattan community. It is a strong voice for improving the lives of those living in the community. Alianza is consulted frequently by the major institutions and looked at as a partner with the capacity to deliver. A visible sign of the growth of this organization is apparent by looking at its facility. The community health worker chapter (chapter 3) described the origins of the organization in 1987 and how its first home required them to chase out drug addicts. Today, Alianza is completing the construction of a new six-story building in the midst of the Columbia University Medical Center campus. The university helped Alianza by leasing it the land for its new facility on Columbia property and will rent space from Alianza. This is quite a change—going from an organization that was wary of the institutions to one that is able to interact in a positive way with the major institutions in northern Manhattan. Alianza continues to collaborate with the Mailman School of Public Health to develop the field of community health workers. Alianza is a credible source in northern Manhattan and has grown to be recognized locally and nationally.

The Thelma C. Davidson Adair Medical and Dental Center (chapter 13) has been approved by New York State to become part of the Ryan network, a Public Health Section 330 Community Health Center organization. Established in 2001 with a mission to provide medical and dental services to low-income people, the Adair Center will continue to serve the Harlem community as part of this network which receives ongoing federal and state support for services provided. In fact, the handoff from Columbia to Ryan happened on July 1, 2009, without a break in service.

The Columbia University College of Dental Medicine and the Harlem Hospital Dental Service collaborated on other programs beyond building the Community DentCare network (chapter 11) and the planning of the Thelma C. Davidson Adair Medical/Dental Center. For example, both partners recognized the need for the Harlem community to have a cadre of African American dental specialists on the hospital staff and to serve on the faculty of the College of Dental Medicine. The Dental Service at Harlem prior to establishing this special program to train underrepresented minority specialists had no trained dental specialists, making it impossible for the service to provide comprehensive care to the population it serves. As the dental safety net provider in Harlem and anchor for the Community DentCare program in Harlem, it was critical to train such specialists. The College of Dentistry recognized that it needed to recruit and train underrepresented minority faculty in order for it to help the profession of dentistry attract minorities into its field and to provide leadership for initiatives to train diverse practitioners for the demographic shift in the country toward a diverse population. The college and the hospital created a program that over a ten- to twelve-year period trained twenty-one dentists in six specialty fields (periodontics, endondontics, orthodontics, prosthodontics, pediatric dentistry, and public health). All of the individuals accepted into the program were from the staff of Harlem Hospital. The university provided free tuition, and the hospital continued to pay a salary because of the compelling needs to build the dental staff at Harlem and bring more minorities onto the college faculty. The outcome of this program has been extraordinary. Fifteen of the twenty-one dentists who completed this program hold academic appointments, four full time at Columbia, one full time at Case Western Reserve, and ten others part time at Columbia. One of the four full-time faculty members at Columbia is the head of his specialty division and another is an associate dean. Nine of the graduates hold joint appointments at the Harlem Hospital, and two are full time at the hospital. These individuals have enabled the Harlem Hospital Dental Service to provide comprehensive dental care for children and adults. Many are the first African American or Hispanic individuals trained in New York City. The College of Dental Medicine continues to grow the Community DentCare network, just recently adding a new dental service in a public school in Harlem.

We believe the idea of collaboration works when there is a mutual benefit to the parties involved. The illustrations above and the book chapters demonstrate that collaboration for the betterment of society trumps narrow interests. Nonprofit, community-based organizations and academic health science centers working together can tackle the larger issues confronting society. There are many other examples of how the collaborators cited in this book have continued on in other ways to collaborate to improve the well-being in the community. One final noteworthy example recently under way is an organized effort by New York Presbyterian Hospital and the Columbia University Medical Center called the Washington Heights Initiative. The initiative is designed to better align the academic health center's delivery system in northern Manhattan by coordinating care with community providers and to further improve relations with community physicians, organizations, and patients. Some of the initiative's aims, such as undertaking strategic planning to enhance primary care and the patient-centered medical home concept and strategic planning for chronic disease management and preventive interventions, will further the work begun by the NMCVC. Whether this new Hospital-Academic Medical Center effort is a direct or indirect result of the path laid down by the decade of Community Voices will never be completely known, but many of those whose vision and tireless work contributed to NMCVC can be credited for the progress seen today as proponents of health reform through linking with communities to improve health and health outcomes.

There has been a renaissance in northern Manhattan. The Northern Manhattan Community Voices Collaborative initiative came around at the right time to help fuel that renaissance. Those who were part of this initiative have taken the spirit of it in new directions and spawned new efforts of collaboration between the institutions and the community for improvement. That is not to say, however, that the institutions that are located in northern Manhattan and their surrounding community no longer disagree on issues. They do, but there remains a greater sensitivity on the part of both that it is important to work out differences through dialogue, communication, and continuing the process of building trusting relationships.

Acronyms Used in the Book

ABC	Asthma Basics for Children Inititative
CARE	Care Coordination, Advocacy, Reconnaissance, and Education
CBO	community-based organization
CBPR	Community Based Participatory Research
CDC	Centers for Disease Control
CDM	College of Dental Medicine
CHP	Child Health Plus
CHW	community health worker
CSAT	Center for Substance Abuse Treatment
CUMC	Columbia University Medical Center
DOHMH	Department of Health and Mental Hygiene
FQHC	Federally Qualified Health Center
GNYHA	Greater New York Hospital Association
HITE	Health Information Tool for Empowerment
HP/DP	Health Promotion and Disease Prevention
HUD	Housing and Urban Development
NMCVC	Northern Manhattan Community Voices Collaborative
NMIC	Northern Manhattan Improvement Corporation
NMIP	Northern Manhattan Immunization Partnership
NMMHC	Northern Manhattan Mental Health Council
NYPH	New York Presbyterian Hospital

OASAS	Office of Alcohol and Substance Abuse Services
PACE	Physician Asthma Care Education Program
PCDC	Primary Care Development Corporation
SASA	Salud a Su Alcance
SASA–DMP	Salud a Su Alcance Diabetes Management Program
SASA–PAP	Salud a Su Alcance Pharmacy Assistance Program
SNP	Special Needs Plan
TBC	Target Behavioral Care
WEP	Welfare Employment Program
WH/I	Washington Heights/Inwood
WIC	Special Supplemental Nutrition Program for Women, Infants, and Children

List of Contributors

Editors

Allan J. Formicola is Professor emeritus of Dentistry and Dean emeritus of the Columbia University College of Dental Medicine (1978–2001). He is the founder of the Center for Community Health Partnerships, which merged into the Center for Family and Community Medicine at Columbia University. Formicola brought together the collaboration between Columbia University Medical Center, Alianza Dominicana, and Harlem Hospital Medical Center to establish the Northern Manhattan Community Voices Collaborative. Under his leadership as Dean of the College of Dental Medicine, the Community DentCare network was developed and the Thelma C. Davidson Adair Medical/Dental Center was established. He currently directs or codirects a number of national foundation projects dealing with oral health disparities and lack of access to dental care.

Lourdes Hernández-Cordero is an Assistant Professor of Clinical Sociomedical Sciences at the Columbia University Mailman School of Public Health. She was the former and final Executive Director for the Northern Manhattan Community Voices Collaborative. During her training in public health, she received a Community Voices Scholars scholarship and authored the mental health report titled *Mental Health: The Neglected Epidemic*. Hernández-Cordero currently facilitates a number of community-based research and intervention projects that draw on the relationships developed during her tenure at the collaborative.

Gail C. Christopher (foreword) is Vice President for Programs at the W. K. Kellogg Foundation. She serves on the executive team that provides overall direction and leadership for the Kellogg Foundation and provides leadership for the Food, Health & Well-Being and Racial Equity programs. She is a nationally recognized leader in health policy, with particular expertise and experience in the issues related to social determinants of health, health disparities, and public policy issues of concern to African Americans and other minority populations. A prolific writer and presenter, she is the author or coauthor of three books, a monthly column in the *Federal Times*, and more than 250 articles, presentations, and publications.

Nancy Bruning lives and works in northern Manhattan. She has authored or co-authored over twenty-five books on health and fitness, wellness, arts and culture, and the environment and has edited and contributed to many more. She has also worked as a researcher and program consultant for the New York Academy of Medicine, the Mailman School of Public Health, and the Immigration and Health Initiative at Hunter. Bruning is the managing editor for this volume.

Chapter Authors

David Albert is Director of Community Health and Associate Professor of Clinical Dentistry and Public Health at the Columbia University School of Dental and Oral Surgery and the Joseph Mailman School of Public Health at Columbia University. Albert is currently co-Principal Investigator of a National Institutes of Health research study that is investigating the effectiveness of tobacco cessation counseling by dental clinicians in public health settings. He is a co-investigator in the Manhattan Tobacco Cessation Center, a New York State Department of Health project. Albert developed and directed the Advanced Education in General Dentistry program at Columbia University. He implemented the dental service of the Ambulatory Care Network of Presbyterian Hospital and now directs the Fort Washington Dental Service, where he maintains a geriatric dental practice within the community of Washington Heights/Inwood in northern Manhattan.

Yisel Alonzo was the Assistant Program Director for the Northern Manhattan Community Voices Collaborative. In that role, she developed strategic alliances with community-based organizations, institutions, and public and private agencies. She successfully carried out the HITE and Healthy Choices projects. Alonzo is a Health Education Specialist with certification from the National Commission for Health Education Credentialing Inc.

Mario Drummonds is the Executive Director/CEO of the Northern Manhattan Perinatal Partnership, Inc., a Harlem-based maternal and child health agency working to improve the health status of pregnant and parenting women in northern Manhattan. He is an expert in the areas of program administration and planning, lectures on the theory and practice of building a public health social movement locally to decrease racial disparities in birth outcomes, and assists other Healthy Start projects in the nation to develop sustainability strategies and prepare competitive Healthy Start applications. He is a member of the faculty of U.S. Health Resources and Services Administration's Quality Institute and a faculty member of the National Healthy Start Association Leadership Institute. The administration has designated the Central Harlem Healthy Start program as a center of excellence in maternal and child health service delivery while achieving outstanding birth outcomes.

Sally Findley is Professor of Clinical Population and Family Health and Clinical Sociomedical Sciences (in Pediatrics), Mailman School of Public Health, Columbia University; a founding member of the Northern Manhattan Community Voices Collaborative; a member of the steering committee; evaluation director for the collaborative; and cochair of the Health Promotion and Disease Prevention working group. She collaborated with Alianza Dominicana in establishing and strengthening a training program for facilitated enrollers for the child health insurance program and has continued to collaborate with Alianza in developing programs to train community health workers. Findley worked with community partners to establish the Northern Manhattan Start Right Coalition and the Northern Manhattan Asthma Basics for Children Initiative. She continues to work with these community partners, further adapting the community health worker model of Northern Manhattan Community Voices Collaborative to activities to reduce childhood obesity and cardiovascular risk. She serves on the board of directors for the Community Health Worker Network of New York City.

Laura Frye is a Management Consultant at Nonprofit Consulting Services, a program of Public Health Solutions. Frye builds the capacity of community-based organizations through trainings and one-on-one technical assistance in the areas of program planning, staff supervision, behavioral sciences, and monitoring and evaluation. She also develops curriculum and trains agencies on implementing effective behavioral interventions for HIV prevention. Prior to joining Public Health Solutions, Frye conducted independent research in Morocco on the health ramifications of legal changes in the country's Family Code under a Fulbright Scholarship. She has also worked on reproductive health issues in El Salvador and Thailand.

Sandra Harris is currently the Assistant Vice President for Government and Community Affairs at Columbia University Medical Center. In her capacity, she continues to foster collaborative partnerships between university- and community-based organization around health care issues impacting residents in the Washington Heights/Inwood community. Harris has worked in that community for the past twenty years. During this time, she has worked with community organizations, public officials, services providers, and residents. In 1998 she joined Columbia University Medical Center as Executive Director for the Northern Manhattan Community Voices Collaborative.

Matilde Irigoyen is Chair of the Department of Pediatrics and Adolescent Medicine at Albert Einstein Medical Center in Philadelphia. Previously, Irigoyen was Professor of Clinical Pediatrics and Population and Family Health and Director of General Pediatrics at Columbia University. She completed residency and fellowship at Mount Sinai Medical Center in New York. As a strong advocate for childhood immunization, Irigoyen has worked with multiple coalitions in New York City.

Kathleen Klink is the Director of the Center for Family and Community Medicine at Columbia University. Klink completed service in the office of Senator Hillary Rodham Clinton as a Robert Wood Johnson Health Policy Fellow in December 2008, where she worked with senior health staff in evaluating and formulating legislation and led meetings with constituent groups, government, and other interested parties regarding health policy issues. Prior to arriving at Columbia, she was the Medical Director at the Coney Island Community Health Center, where she spearheaded community initiatives and initiated an innovative quality assurance program. As Associate Director for Family Medicine, she developed the curriculum for the first family medicine residency training program at Columbia University Medical Center/New York Presbyterian Hospital. Recently she led the expansion of the Center for Family and Community Medicine, which serves Washington Heights/Inwood, to enhance its research and development missions.

Harris K. (Ken) Lampert is Chief of Ambulatory Care and Associate Medical Director at Lincoln Medical and Mental Health Center and was the President and CEO of Community Premier Plus, Inc. (1996–2007), a nonprofit managed care plan serving Medicaid and uninsured clients. He is board certified in internal medicine and maintained a primary care practice for many years. He was an Assistant Professor of Clinical Medicine at the College of Physicians and Surgeons of Columbia University (1995–2007) and served as Chair of the New York State Coalition of Prepaid Health Services Plans (2003–2006).

Anita Lee is the founder and President of ALMS Healthcare Management, Inc., a private company that enhances the impact of nonprofit organizations serving low-income communities through administrative, governance, fund-raising, and program development support. In 2007 she cofounded NYCRx, a nonprofit organization that implements low-cost pharmaceutical access solutions for safety net providers, and in 2002 she founded the Salud A Su Alcance Pharmacy Assistance Program at New York Presbyterian Hospital, which helps uninsured patients to access free medicine. As Director of Network Development for Continuum Health Partners from 1998 to 2001, Lee expanded the capacity of many Federally Qualified Health Centers by cultivating collaborative partnerships between the centers and hospital systems. She has an expansive track record of building community capacity and infrastructure to improve health outcomes and has extensive experience in developing and managing health care programs, organizations, and coalitions. She has devoted her professional life to improving health care access and the quality of care for the uninsured and underinsured.

Maria Lizardo has been working at Northern Manhattan Improvement Corporation since 1998 as the Director of Social Services. Lizardo is responsible for the following programs: Health Care Access, Lead Poisoning Prevention Program, Asthma Program, Domestic Violence Program, Single Stop Benefits Screening and Access, and Case Management Services. Lizardo has been an active participant representing the Northern Manhattan Improvement Corporation on the Asthma Basics for Children Coalition since its inception under the Northern Manhattan Community Voices Collaborative.

Rosa Madera-Reese is the Community Health Coordinator for the Asthma Basics for Children Program established under the Northern Manhattan Community Voices Collaborative. Her primary responsibilities include implementing the ashthma program in designated Head Start/day care and school settings in Washington Heights and Harlem.

Stephen Marshall is the Associate Dean for Extramural Programs at the Columbia University College of Dental Medicine. Since 1988 he has held various position at the college, including Acting Director for the Division of Community Health, Director of Clinical Business Affairs and Managed Care, Chair of the Quality Assurance Committee, and Assistant Dean for Patient Care Programs. He was instrumental in establishing the Community DentCare program and played a pivotal role in administering the Thelma C. Davidson Adair Mental/Dental Center in Harlem. He is currently responsible for the Community DentCare program, the ElderSmile program, hospital relationships, dental plans, and continuing education programs.

Jacqueline Martínez is the Senior Program Director at the New York State Health Foundation. She serves as a key advisor to the president and CEO and leads two of the foundation's program areas. Prior to joining the foundation, Martínez served as the Executive Director for the Northern Manhattan Community Voices Collaborative, where she implemented and evaluated health programs in obesity prevention, mental health, case management, and childhood asthma. Under the leadership of the National Community Voices Collaborative, she worked to mobilize national, state, and local resources to promote policy changes to address the health care concerns addressed by the program. Martínez has also served as program manager for Alianza Dominicana and was a National Institutes of Health Fellow in Yucatan, Mexico, and an Assistant Coordinator for Beginning with Children, a Brooklyn-based charter school. She has served as Adjunct Professor of Sociology at the Borough of Manhattan Community College, Board Director of the Institute for Civic Leadership, and Board Member of the National Alliance on Mental Illness–New York City Metro.

James McIntosh is currently an Oral Health Community Activist in Harlem. He served as the Director for the Department of Dentistry at the Harlem Hospital Center for over twenty years. He helped to develop the collaboration between the hospital and the College of Dental Medicine at Columbia University, which significantly increased the oral health services that were delivered to the Harlem community. Included in the numerous other accomplishments during his tenure as Director, McIntosh spearheaded the development of the Minority Postgraduate Specialty Training Program, which allowed twenty-three African American graduates from the Harlem Hospital Center general practice dental residency program to matriculate into numerous College of Dental Medicine dental specialty training programs. Most of the graduates returned to teach and practice their disciplines in the community.

Miriam Mejía is the Deputy Director at Alianza Dominicana and facilitated many of the initiatives between Alianza and Columbia described in this book. A native of the Dominican Republic, she studied statistics and sociology at the Universidad Autonoma de Santo Domingo in the nation's capital. Subsequently, she dedicated ten years of her life to conducting sociological investigations on the status of women in her country. She has published five books, the latest of which is *Aristas Ancestrales*, a book of poems.

Dennis Mitchell is the Associate Dean for Diversity and Multicultural Affairs at the Columbia University College of Dental Medicine and responsible for the dental schools' diversity initiatives targeted for training, faculty development, and student enrollment. Mitchell served as the Director of the Harlem component of the

Community DentCare network and the Director of Research and Community Dentistry at the Harlem Hospital Center Department of Dentistry for nine years. Mitchell was the co-Principal Investigator for the Columbia University site of the National Institutes of Health–funded Obstetrics and Periodontal Therapy multi-center randomized clinical trial investigating the effects of periodontal therapy on preterm birth. His wide-ranging professional activities have led to his selection for numerous speaking engagements.

Benjamin Ortiz is currently Assistant Professor of Clinical Pediatrics and Clinical Population and Family Health, Columbia University College of Physicians and Surgeons and Mailman School of Public Health, and Assistant Attending Physician, Harlem Hospital Center, Department of Pediatrics. His primary role is as general pediatrician for the children of central and East Harlem, Washington Heights, and the South Bronx who receive pediatric care in the Harlem Hospital Pediatric Ambulatory Center. Additionally, he is co-Principal Investigator and Assistant Medical Director of the Harlem Children's Zone Asthma Initiative, co-Principal Investigator for the Northern Manhattan Asthma Basics for Children Initiative, and Principal Investigator for the Childhood Obesity Prevention and Treatment program at Harlem Hospital.

Martin Ovalles became a Tobacco Cessation Specialist and a Clinical Coordinator for the Tobacco Cessation Clinic at the College of Dental Medicine. For several years he has been involved with research on type-2 diabetes in adolescents and youth at the Naomi Berrie Diabetes Center at Columbia University Medical Center.

Moisés Pérez is founder and executive director of Alianza Dominicana, the largest community agency for Dominicans in the United States. Alianza Dominicana began in a public housing storefront in 1986 and has since opened eight other offices in the Washington Heights, Inwood, central Harlem, and Bronx communities. The non-profit organization has created nationally recognized programs in youth development, family-centered substance abuse treatment, mental health, HIV/AIDS education and prevention, health promotion, and child abuse prevention. Pérez is a founding member of the Hispanic Federation of New York City, the Agenda for Children Tomorrow, and Northern Manhattan Collaborates, a broad-based planning group serving Harlem and Washington Heights. His leadership and commitment to the development of underserved communities have led to widespread recognition.

Cheryl Ragonesi is a Licensed Clinical Social Worker with interest and expertise in substance abuse counseling, community organizing, palliative care, geriatrics, program administration, and teaching. She is currently working at Continuum Hospice Care of New York and teaching at the Columbia University College of Dental Medicine.

Martha Sánchez was born and raised in Harlem in New York City. She has been working for over thirty years as a community organizer, public health advocate, and health educator in programs addressing the elimination of health disparities. Her work includes a focus on improving the health status of women, children, and families.

Daniel F. Seidman is a member of the Columbia University Behavioral Medicine Faculty and a practicing psychotherapist. His research interests include developing innovative approaches to assist underserved and highly addicted smokers. He is coeditor and contributing author to the book *Helping the Hard-Core Smoker: A Clinician's Guide* (Lawrence Erlbaum, 1999). He is also author of the book *Smoke-free in 30 Days* (Touchstone/Fireside Simon & Schuster, 2010), based on a program featured on the *Oprah Winfrey Show* in January 2008. Seidman has a Ph.D. degree from Columbia University in clinical psychology.

Susan Sturm is the George M. Jaffin Professor of Law and Social Responsibility at Columbia Law School, where her principal areas of teaching and research include institutional change, structural inequality in employment and higher education, employment discrimination, public law remedies, conflict resolution, and civil procedure. She is the founding Director of the Center for Institutional and Social Change at the Law School, www.groundshift.org, and a founding member of the Presidential Advisory Committee on Diversity Initiatives at Columbia. She has published numerous articles and books on "the architecture of inclusion," institutional change, transformative leadership, workplace equality, legal education, and inclusion and diversity in higher education, which are available on her website at www2.law .columbia.edu/ssturm/. She is one of the architects of the national conference on The Future of Diversity and Opportunity in Higher Education. She is also the Principal Investigator for grants from the Ford Foundation, Harvard University, and the Kirwan Institute, awarded to develop the architecture of inclusion in higher education.

Gloria Thomas has been a Program Coordinator for the Northern Manhattan Asthma Basics for Children Initiative at the Mailman School of Public Health, Columbia University, since 2002. She coordinates the development, implementation, expansion, and day-to-day operations of the initiative, which aim is to help families better manage their children's asthma. She has also worked as a Program Coordinator in various HIV/AIDS clinical trials at Harlem Hospital Medical Center.

Index

288

Index